Fourth Edition

UNIPAC 9

Caring for Patients with Chronic Illnesses: Dementia, COPD, and CHF

Joseph W. Shega, MD
University of Chicago
Chicago, IL

Stacie K. Levine, MD
University of Chicago
Chicago, IL

Reviewed by
Solomon Liao, MD FAAHPM
University of California–Irvine
Irvine, CA

Edited by
C. Porter Storey, Jr., MD FACP FAAHPM
Colorado Permanente Medical Group
Executive Vice President
American Academy of Hospice and Palliative
  Medicine
Boulder, CO

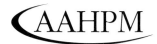

American Academy of Hospice and Palliative Medicine
4700 W. Lake Avenue
Glenview, IL 60025-1485
aahpm.org | PalliativeDoctors.org

© 2012 American Academy of Hospice and Palliative Medicine
First edition published 1997 (*UNIPAC 9* was not included with the first edition)
Second edition published 2003 (*UNIPAC 9* was not included with the second edition)
Third edition published 2008

Publishing Staff
Julie Bruno, Senior Education Manager
Angie Forbes, Education Manager
Jerrod Liveoak, Senior Managing Editor
Katie Macaluso, Managing Editor
Monica Piotrowski, Assistant Editor
Sonya Jones, Senior Designer
Stephanie Euzebio, Graphic Designer
Cover design and page layout by Stephanie Euzebio

ISBN 978-1-889296-49-4

Contents

Tables

Figures

Acknowledgments

The editor, authors, contributors, and the American Academy of Hospice and Palliative Medicine are deeply grateful to all who have participated in the development of this component of the *UNIPAC: A Resource for Hospice and Palliative Care Professionals* self-study program. The expertise of the contributors and reviewers involved in the previous and current edition of the *UNIPACs* has greatly improved their value and contents. Our special thanks are extended to the pharmacist reviewer for *UNIPAC 9*, James B. Ray, PharmD; the reviewer for the *UNIPAC 9 amplifire* confidence-based learning module, Dominic F. Glorioso, DO; Jay Thomas, MD PhD, and Kathleen McGrady, MD MS MA FAAHPM, for their reviews of the previous edition of *UNIPAC 9*; and Tasnim Sinuff, MD PhD FRCPC; Robert Horton, MD FCPF; and Paul Hernandez, MDCM FRCPC, for their contributions to the article previously published in the *Journal of Palliative Medicine* that served as the basis for the chapter in this book titled "Chronic Obstructive Pulmonary Disease."

Continuing Medical Education

Purpose
A *UNIPAC* is a packet of information formatted as an independent-study program. It includes practical clinical scenarios to orient the reader to the material, educational content, and references. This independent-study program is intended for healthcare providers who are interested in incorporating the principles of hospice and palliative medicine into their daily practice. It is designed to increase competence in palliative care interventions for improving a patient's quality of life. Specific, practical information is presented to help physicians and other practitioners assess and manage selected problems. After reading the *UNIPAC*, practitioners are encouraged to complete a separate online confidence-based learning module. Physicians may only obtain *AMA PRA Category 1 Credits*™ by completing this module.

Learning Objectives
Upon completion of this continuing medical education (CME) program, a physician should be better able to

Dementia
- identify the most common etiologies of dementia and their pathogenesis in the United States
- understand the prevalence of dementia in the United States and its age-related variation
- describe the typical disease course for a person with Alzheimer's dementia
- describe the currently available pharmacologic therapies for the treatment of Alzheimer's disease, including their mechanisms of action, indications, and common side effects
- develop a strategy to assess pain in people with mild-to-moderate and severe-to-end-stage dementia
- list the behavioral and psychological symptoms of dementia (BPSD)
- describe the difference between depression and apathy and understand the unique features of depression in people with dementia, including prevalence, alternative presentations, and treatment options
- list the most commonly used atypical antipsychotics, with dosage recommendations and possible adverse effects
- identify contributing causes to agitation in people with dementia
- recognize frequent complications in patients with end-stage dementia and an approach to their treatment
- review hospice eligibility guidelines for dementia and summarize their limitations
- appreciate the impact of caregiving on people with dementia compared to other life-limiting illnesses.

Chronic Obstructive Pulmonary Disease (COPD)
- list the most common etiologies, prevalence, burden, and mortality of COPD
- describe the disease trajectory for patients with COPD

- describe the neurophysiology of dyspnea
- demonstrate the assessment and treatment of COPD and dyspnea, including pharmacologic approaches, oxygen, opioids, and nonpharmacologic approaches
- discuss the indications for noninvasive ventilation (NIV) for patients with end-stage COPD
- refer appropriate patients with COPD to palliative care and hospice
- communicate effectively with patients about end-of-life (EOL) care options for patients with COPD
- describe the impact of anxiety and depression on patients with COPD
- educate patients and families on home care and self-management of COPD.

Congestive Heart Failure (CHF)
- list CHF classifications (New York Heart Association [NYHA] class and American College of Cardiology/American Heart Association [ACC/AHA] staging)
- describe the disease course and illness trajectory in CHF
- discuss when to initiate palliative care for CHF
- list difficulties in predicting prognosis in CHF
- discuss the prognosis for a patient with CHF, including the differences in prognosis and therapies for patients with preserved ejection fraction
- describe medical and invasive therapies for CHF and how they translate to the palliative care setting
- apply strategies for dosing of sedating medications for CHF
- discuss symptom burden in CHF
- describe when it is appropriate to refer patients with CHF to hospice.

Disclosure

In accordance with the Accreditation Council for Continuing Medical Education's Standards for Commercial Support, all CME providers are required to disclose to the activity audience the relevant financial relationships of the planners, reviewers, and authors involved in the development of CME content. An individual has a relevant financial relationship if he or she has a financial relationship in any amount occurring in the last 12 months with a commercial interest whose products or services are discussed in the CME activity content over which the individual has control. AAHPM requires that all relevant financial relationships be resolved prior to planning or participating in the activity. **The authors, editor, and reviewers for this module have disclosed no relevant financial relationships.**

Term of Offering

The release date for the *UNIPAC 9 **amplifire*** module is April 1, 2012, and the expiration date is March 31, 2015.

Dementia

Dementia is an acquired loss of memory that is substantial enough to interfere with everyday functioning plus impairment of at least one other cognitive domain. Given its prolonged course and associated behavioral and psychological symptoms, the care of people with dementia presents numerous opportunities to integrate palliative care from diagnosis to end of life (EOL). Each stage of the disease (mild, moderate, severe, and end stage) reflects a decline in cognitive and functional abilities for which palliative interventions can improve outcomes and quality of life (QOL). With the increasing prevalence of dementia, palliative medicine clinicians will care for increasing numbers of patients with dementia either as a primary diagnosis or as a condition that coexists with another life-limiting condition. In addition to caring for patients, clinicians also need to tend to caregivers' well-being because they play a vital role in the health of people with dementia. Taken together, a palliative model focuses on both the patient and caregiver's physical, psychological, social, and spiritual care. The nature and focus of care is modified over time as a patient's memory loss and functional dependence progress and caregivers' roles change.

Diagnosis and Meaningful Subtypes

Table 1 displays some of the more common etiologies of dementia for which an accurate clinical diagnosis relies on strict and validated criteria. During the past decade, characteristic symptoms of the various subtypes of dementia have been found to correspond with pathological changes in the brain (eg, protein deposition, ischemia).[1] These changes in the brain, along with an individual's life experiences and comorbid conditions, influence prognosis, symptomatology, treatment, and expected disease course. As a dementia progresses, clinical symptoms become remarkably similar among the various subtypes, making an etiology-based diagnosis more difficult. In the more advanced stages of dementia, a patient's prognosis, symptoms, and treatment decisions overlap considerably, resulting in a more consistent management approach.

Memory changes that occur with advanced age can be conceptualized as existing on a continuum: normal changes, mild cognitive impairment, and dementia. For example, it is normal for older adults to need more time to learn new information, but older adults can retain the same amount of information as younger people.[2] Patients with mild cognitive impairment exhibit abnormalities

Table 1. Most Common Etiologies of Dementia in the United States

Dementia Diagnosis	Relative Frequency	Pathophysiology
Alzheimer's disease (AD)	35%	Beta-amyloid plaques and neurofibrillary tangles (tau)
Mixed (vascular disease and AD)	15%	Combination of AD and vascular disease
Lewy body dementia	15%	Alpha-synuclein protein
Vascular dementia	10%	Cortical infarcts, subcortical infarcts, and leukoaraiosis
Frontotemporal dementia (Pick's disease)	5%	Tau protein

Note. Studies indicate that 55% to 70% of dementia cases have a significant component of AD that often coexists with Lewy body dementia and vascular dementia.

apraxia - difficulty articulating
aphasia - can't comprehend/or formulate language

in memory or one other cognitive domain (ie, aphasia, agnosia, apraxia, executive functioning). Other areas of cognition, however, remain intact, and the cognitive deficit does not impair functional abilities. The presence of mild cognitive impairment puts people at high risk for developing dementia over the next several years.[3] Although many types of dementia exist, most patients with dementia have Alzheimer's Disease (AD), vascular dementia, Lewy body dementia, or some combination of these conditions.[4]

AD is the most common cause of dementia in the United States, with a molecular pathogenesis of protein deposition—namely, beta-amyloid plaques and neurofibrillary tangles (tau).[5] The hippocampus and neocortex are the primary affected sites that translate into clinical manifestations of the disease. A clinical diagnosis using validated criteria is correct more than 85% of the time at postmortem examination.[6] The *Diagnostic and Statistical Manual of Mental Disorders*, 4th Edition, Text Revision (DSM-IV-TR) criteria for AD are memory impairment and at least one other cognitive disturbance, such as aphasia, agnosia, apraxia, or executive functioning.[7] The cognitive dysfunction must be severe enough to impair social or occupational functioning and cannot be attributed to another cognitive disorder.[8]

One of the first symptoms of AD is memory loss, particularly, difficulty encoding new memories. As the disease progresses, patients begin to experience disorganized thoughts, confusion, and disorientation. At the same time, affected people begin to have language difficulties, such as substituting words and forgetting the names of objects. Executive functioning also becomes impaired, which results in impaired judgment. In addition to cognitive decline, noncognitive behavioral and psychological symptoms including agitation, psychosis, and mood disorders (predominantly depression) frequently develop.[9]

The Alzheimer's Association and National Institutes of Health have proposed modifying AD diagnostic criteria. This modification includes updated criteria for AD, the designation of mild cognitive impairment likely attributable to AD, and new criteria for people with evidence of preclinical disease. The revised guidelines are intended to incorporate significant scientific advances. These advances include the application of biomarkers obtained from cerebrospinal fluid and the application of newer neuroimaging techniques.[10] The former builds upon evidence that early amyloid deposition in the brain (low cerebrospinal fluid amyloid beta-1-42) leads to neuronal damage (high cerebrospinal fluid tau) and subsequent neurodegeneration (loss of neuronal tissue). Low cerebrospinal fluid of amyloid and high tau indicate the development or presence of AD. The latter incorporates structural and functional imaging to identify changes within the brain suggestive of the presence or evolution (preclinical stage) of AD.[11] Tracers developed for positron emission tomography (PET) to assess for amyloid deposits in vivo, such as Pittsburgh compound B, serve as an example of imaging to detect AD's preclinical stage. Amyloid deposits evident on scan in cognitively intact people have been found to predict a higher risk for developing AD years after the scan.

Vascular dementia is the second most common form of dementia in the United States.[12] The etiology of neuronal loss or dysfunction causing vascular cognitive impairment includes cortical infarcts, subcortical infarcts, and leukoaraiosis (thinning of the cerebral white matter).[13,14] The manifestations of cognitive loss are variable and depend on the location and extent of the underlying lesions. Vascular dementia and AD often coexist; the presence of vascular disease appears to predispose the clinical expression of AD, especially among older adults.[15]

agnosia - lose ability to comprehend/ recognize meaning of objects

Lewy body dementia, another frequent cause of cognitive dysfunction, occurs as a result of alpha-synuclein protein deposition in the cortex and subcortex. Patients exhibit memory loss and deficits in attention, executive functioning, and visuospatial ability.[16,17] A diagnosis of Lewy body dementia includes the presence of core and suggestive features. The core features of the disease include fluctuating cognition with pronounced variations in attention and alertness, recurrent visual hallucinations that are typically well formed and detailed, and spontaneous features of parkinsonism. Suggestive features of the disease include rapid eye movement (REM) sleep behavior disorder, severe neuroleptic sensitivity, and low-dopamine transporter uptake in the basal ganglia on functional imaging. Supportive features such as repeated falls and syncope, transient and unexplained loss of consciousness, and severe autonomic dysfunction are commonly present but lack diagnostic specificity. The presence of Lewy body dementia and parkinsonian symptoms should occur around the same time to differentiate between people with Lewy body dementia and those with Parkinson's disease (PD) who eventually develop dementia years after diagnosis.

Current recommendations for diagnostic testing include screening for vitamin B_{12} deficiency and thyroid disorders, which, if present, may contribute to additional morbidity. Routine screening for syphilis is generally not recommended unless the patient represents a population with a high prevalence of the disease. Physicians should consider neuroimaging if dementia presents with atypical features or if a clinician determines the need based on a history of falls, a focal neurologic examination, or other factors. Although reversible causes of dementia are rare, consideration of potential contributors to cognitive loss (eg, metabolic disorders, drugs, medications, toxins, hepatic disease, kidney disease, vitamin deficiencies, endocrinopathies), psychiatric disease (especially depression), and infectious diseases (eg, acquired immune deficiency syndrome, syphilis, Lyme disease) may lead to discovery of additional morbidities associated with cognitive loss. Screening for additional contributors is individualized based on the patient's history and physical examination.

Epidemiology

Age is the greatest risk factor for dementia; its incidence and prevalence increase dramatically in those older than 65 years. Specifically, AD affects 2% to 3% of people older than 65 years and doubles in incidence for every 5 years of age thereafter. As a result, AD prevalence approaches 50% among those older than 85 years.[18] In a 2010 study conducted by the Alzheimer's Association, more than 5 million people in the United States were reported to have AD, and a person develops the disease every 72 seconds.[19] Because the population of people older than 65 years is growing, the number of Americans with AD is projected to climb to 8 million by 2030.

The rate of deaths attributable to AD continues to rise dramatically. AD is the fifth leading cause of death for people 65 years and older. According to the Centers for Disease Control and Prevention (CDC), AD deaths rose by 46% between 2000 and 2006, whereas deaths from heart disease, cerebrovascular disease, and many malignancies declined during the same period.[19]

People with AD often have coexisting morbidities including hypertension, heart disease, arthritis, diabetes, peripheral vascular disease, and COPD.[20] Consequently, in addition to the cognitive symptoms of AD, patients frequently experience symptoms such as shortness of breath, depression, and pain.[21] As dementia progresses, identifying these physical and psychological conditions becomes challenging, and clinicians need to combine evaluations of caregiver reports and direct observation to optimally assess a patient's well-being.

The financial burden of caring for a person with AD falls on caregivers, employers, and society. The 2010 *Alzheimer's Disease Facts and Figures*, published by the Alzheimer's Association, summarizes the economic impact of dementia in the United States.[19] The direct and indirect cost of AD and other dementias amounts to more than $172 billion annually and does not include the contributions of unpaid caregivers. Caregivers of patients with dementia cost employers $6.5 billion annually in lost productivity, missed work, and replacement workers. In 2005 unpaid caregivers provided almost $83 billion worth of services. Healthcare costs are significantly higher for patients with dementia, and this cost rises substantially as the severity of the condition increases.

CLINICAL SITUATION

Margaret

Margaret is an 80-year-old woman with arthritis who is brought into a physician's office by her 60-year-old son, Robert, who has concerns about her memory. Margaret is widowed and lives alone in a senior citizen housing development. Margaret's neighbor called Robert, who resides in a different state, because her phone service had been discontinued as a result of several unpaid bills. Other neighbors had noticed Margaret appearing "lost" in the supermarket parking lot on multiple occasions and needing help finding her car. Upon visiting his mother, Robert noticed she had posted several reminder notes throughout her apartment and pots with burned food were sitting in her sink.

When asked about these concerns Margaret became defensive and said, "I don't know what you are all talking about. I am not crazy!" Although she has been very irritable, she does not have any symptoms of depression, delusions, or hallucinations. She does not drink alcohol, smoke, or use illicit drugs. She is not taking medications and has no other chronic medical conditions. Her physical examination was positive for Myerson's frontal release sign but was otherwise nonfocal. She scored 19 out of 30 on the Mini-Mental State Examination (MMSE; with a college education). Laboratory results revealed a normal B_{12} and thyrotropin. A brain computed tomography (CT) scan showed small-vessel ischemic changes and diffuse atrophy.

Question One

Robert asks, "Does mother have dementia?" The most appropriate response should be

A. "Dementia can really only be diagnosed at autopsy."

B. "It would be unfair to put this label on her without a brain biopsy."

C. "Her symptoms, examination, and labwork all suggest this diagnosis."

D. "We need an MRI and a screen for syphilis to make sure."

Correct Response and Analysis

The best response is C, which recognizes some uncertainty but helps Robert focus on the most likely diagnosis and ways to manage Margaret's care. Although other tests are occasionally useful, there is nothing in Margaret's history or examination to suggest that more comprehensive testing will be useful. Resources should be dedicated to extensive education for Robert about the nature, likely course, and management of this condition and referrals to available resources in the community.

Question Two
What are the most likely causes of Margaret's dementia?

A. AD only

B. Vascular dementia only

C. Mixed dementia (AD and vascular)

D. Frontotemporal dementia

Correct Response and Analysis
The correct response is C. The scenarios of difficulty paying bills, getting lost, and burning pots, as well as irritability, are characteristic features of AD. However, additional neuropsychiatric testing would be needed to rule out primary or concomitant vascular dementia. Frontotemporal dementia is unlikely because it characteristically affects younger adults and presents with behavioral disturbances, affective symptoms, and speech disturbances with intact spatial orientation and praxis.

Question Three
What additional tests would you consider for this patient to better assess the etiology of memory loss?

A. Neuropsychiatric testing

B. Functional imaging

C. Lumbar puncture

D. Sleep study

Correct Response and Analysis
The correct response is A. Neuropsychiatric testing in conjunction with a comprehensive history and physical examination, targeted laboratory testing, and possibly neuroimaging can lead to an accurate clinical diagnosis of dementia in a majority of patients. If atypical symptoms are present, additional testing may be warranted. For example, if frontotemporal dementia is suspected, functional imaging techniques such as single-photon emission CT, which shows decreased frontal blood flow, and PET scanning, which shows decreased cortical metabolism in frontotemporal regions, can be helpful. A lumbar puncture may be useful if an AD diagnosis remains uncertain, with low beta-amyloid and high tau being characteristic. Also, if Creutzfeldt-Jakob disease is suspected, protein 14-3-3 in the cerebrospinal fluid is present in more than 90% of typical cases. Finally, a sleep study may be helpful if Lewy body dementia (abnormal REM sleep) is suspected or if sleep apnea is thought to contribute to cognitive dysfunction.

Continued on page 11

Disease Trajectory and Management
Description of Typical Disease Course
AD is a terminal illness for which average life expectancy is 4 to 7 years after diagnosis.[22,23] Age at diagnosis appears to influence median survival; a 2010 study found that when dementia is diagnosed when people are in their 60s, they have a 6- to 7-year average life expectancy, which falls to 1.9 years if the diagnosis occurs at age 90 years or older.[24] Most dementias follow a disease course typical of other chronic illnesses, with gradual deterioration punctuated by substantial cognitive and functional decline, usually as the result of an acute illness.[25,26] During recovery from the acute illness, patients with dementia usually establish a new, lower level of cognitive and physical functioning.[27,28] In the advanced stages of the disease, any downturn—commonly a pneumonia, urinary-tract infection, febrile episode, or eating problem—can become a terminal event.[29-31] In fact, patients with advanced dementia admitted to the hospital with pneumonia or hip fracture had a 6-month mortality rate of 50%, a significantly higher rate than that of cognitively intact controls.[32] Similar to AD, many of the more common causes of dementia including vascular, Lewy body,

and frontotemporal dementias follow a similar disease course.[33] However, more rare causes of dementia such as Huntington's disease and Creutzfeldt-Jakob disease follow a much more rapid course of decline, with a life expectancy of months to a few years from disease onset.

The cognitive and functional decline of patients with AD usually follows a typical pattern.[26,34] Patients with mild dementia experience short-term memory loss along with personality changes and difficulties with some instrumental activities of daily living (IADLs) such as medication management and driving. As dementia progresses to the moderate stage, marked loss of short-term memory occurs, along with a decline in long-term memory. At the same time, patients have difficulty with most IADLs (eg, shopping, meal preparation, housework) and begin to develop difficulty completing complex activities of daily living (ADLs) such as bathing. When dementia is severe, most memory is lost and patients have difficulty with basic ADLs including toileting, dressing, and transferring. At the end stage, patients mutter few intelligible words, become bed bound, and develop progressive dysphagia. At this point, patients have a limited life expectancy and meet hospice eligibility requirements.

Treatment Options: Efficacy, Burdens and Benefits, and Potential Rehabilitation

Pharmacologic

Given the projected increase in the number of people with AD,[19] efforts have been focused on both prevention and delay of onset. To date, no medical interventions have been found that delay the onset of dementia. However, pharmacologic and nonpharmacologic therapies that ameliorate cognitive and functional decline and decrease challenging behaviors are available for people who develop the clinical symptoms of AD. Good medical care necessitates optimal management of coexisting conditions[20] and ensures that prescribed treatments fit within goals of therapy.[35]

Cholinesterase inhibitors and N-methyl-D-aspartate (NMDA) receptor antagonists are the only two classes of medication approved by the US Food and Drug Administration (FDA) for the treatment of Alzheimer's dementia. Cholinergic neurons innervate areas of the brain involved with memory and learning, and many of the core symptoms of AD can be linked to decreases in cholinergic transmission.[36] Cholinesterase inhibitors suppress acetylcholinesterase activity, which degrades acetylcholine in the synaptic cleft. As a result, the synaptic levels of acetylcholine increase, improving neurotransmission and attenuating some of AD's cognitive symptoms.

Cholinesterase inhibitors that are currently available include donepezil, rivastigmine, and galantamine. All three agents are approved by the FDA for the treatment of mild to moderate AD. In addition, donepezil is currently the only cholinesterase inhibitor approved for the treatment of moderate to severe AD. These agents have slightly different mechanisms of action on acetylcholinesterase, but clinical outcomes are remarkably similar (**Table 2**). FDA approval of these agents requires cognitive benefits and demonstrable differences in global impression of change in favor of the study drug. Donepezil is the most widely prescribed acetylcholinesterase inhibitor, probably because of its convenient once-a-day dosing, superior tolerability, and approval for all stages of the disease.[37]

For those with mild to moderate Alzheimer's dementia (ie, patients meet standard diagnostic criteria for AD with MMSE scores of 10 to 26 out of 30, with no other contributing etiology to memory loss), active treatment with cholinesterase inhibitors provides superior cognitive, functional, and behavioral outcomes compared with placebo.[38-40] Cognitive

Table 2. Medications Commonly Used to Treat Alzheimer's Disease

Medication	Mechanism of Action	Disease Severity Indication	Dosage	Side Effects
Donepezil (Aricept)	Reversible acetylcholinesterase inhibitor	Mild to moderate; moderate to severe	5 mg-10 mg/d; 23 mg/d for moderate to severe; start 5 mg at bedtime	Nausea, vomiting, diarrhea (less common); at 23 mg dose, side effects double compared to 10 mg dose
Galantamine (Razadyne, Razadyne ER)	Reversible acetylcholinesterase inhibitor; nicotinic modulation	Mild to moderate	8 mg-24 mg/d; start 4 mg twice daily with meals	Nausea, vomiting, diarrhea, weight loss
Rivastigmine (Exelon)	Pseudoirreversible inhibitor of acetylcholinesterase	Mild to moderate	Oral 6 mg-12 mg/d; start 1.5 mg twice daily. Patch 4.6 mg/d; increase to 9.5 mg/d after 4 weeks	Nausea and vomiting (more common), diarrhea, weight loss, dizziness. Patch has fewer side effects overall but may be associated with pigment changes on skin.
Memantine (Namenda)	Noncompetitive antagonist NMDA receptors	Moderate to severe	20 mg/d; start 5 mg/d	Hypertension, constipation, dizziness, headache. Reduce dose in severe renal impairment

NMDA, N-methyl-D-aspartate.

performance measurement in most of the trials used the Alzheimer's Disease Assessment Scale-Cognitive (ADAS-Cog), a 70-point, 11-item scale that assesses memory, language, orientation, reason, and praxis; a 3-point difference over time is considered clinically significant. In general, 15% to 20% of patients in clinical trials showed marked improvement in cognitive performance (ie, a 7-point change in ADAS-Cog scores over time), and 30% displayed some improvement (ie, a 3-point change in ADAS-Cog scores over time) compared with placebo over 3 to 6 months. The number needed to treat to obtain the clinical benefit was around 4 to 6, depending on the clinical study. Statistically and clinically significant differences in cognitive performance emerged by 12 weeks and persisted until the end of the study (usually 24 weeks). Few of the clinical trials lasted beyond 24 to 36 weeks; however, active treatment continued to be associated with clinically significant benefit compared with placebo in several studies that continued to 1 year.

Studies using donepezil that were designed to specifically assess functional outcomes found that active treatment was associated with a 38% reduction in functional decline, which is defined as an inability to perform one or more ADLs, inability to perform 20% or more of IADLs, or a global worsening in severity of dementia from baseline compared with the placebo group.[41,42] Stated another way, the median time to clinically evident functional decline was 208 days for the placebo group versus 357 days for the donepezil-treated group. The probability of no clinically evident functional decline at 48 weeks was 51% for the donepezil group and 35% for the placebo group.

Neuropsychiatric symptoms may also improve with cholinesterase inhibitor therapy. A meta-analysis of cholinesterase inhibitor trials found that these agents provided a modest benefit that alleviated neuropsychiatric symptoms.[42] The behaviors studied were delusions, hallucinations, agitation, depression, anxiety, euphoria, apathy, disinhibition, irritability, aberrant motor behavior, nighttime behaviors, and appetite and eating disorders. The improvement represents an effect size similar to that of antipsychotic drug trials.[43] A 2007 randomized controlled trial (RCT) that enrolled subjects with AD and refractory agitation who resided in the nursing home setting found donepezil to be no more efficacious than placebo in decreasing these behaviors.[44]

Because functional impairment and behavioral disturbances are associated with an increased risk of nursing home placement for people with Alzheimer's dementia and that cholinesterase inhibitors improve these patients' cognitive, functional, and behavioral outcomes, it has been hypothesized that use of such agents may delay nursing home placement. One study found that donepezil used at higher dosages (10 mg daily) was associated with a 17.5-month delay in nursing home placement. Another study found that cholinesterase inhibitor therapy significantly reduced the risk of nursing home placement by 28% at 12 months and 21% at 18 months; however, by 36 months the risk of nursing home placement was not statistically different between active therapy and placebo. Taken together, it appears that cholinesterase inhibitor therapy may temporarily delay nursing home placement for people with Alzheimer's dementia.[45,46]

Donepezil is the only cholinesterase inhibitor approved for the treatment of moderate to severe AD. Two published double-blind, placebo-controlled, randomized studies found significant benefit with active treatment of 10 mg daily on cognitive, functional, and global impression of change outcomes.[47,48] A 23-mg formulation has received FDA approval for moderate to severe AD. At this higher dose, participants on average had only a two-point improvement on the Severe Impairment Battery (SIB), which was developed to measure cognition in people with moderate to severe dementia (scores range from 0-100)

compared with the 10-mg dose, but participants had about twice the number of side effects, particularly nausea and vomiting, diarrhea, and dizziness.[49]

To date, studies have not included enough hospice-eligible patients to determine whether cholinesterase inhibitors could benefit patients with end-stage dementia. Many experts argue that the likelihood of clinically relevant improvement or disease stabilization in bed-bound, mostly nonverbal patients remains remote. Others argue that patients with end-stage dementia maintain some independent functioning, such as holding up their head without assistance or swallowing food without aspiration, and consequently may benefit from cholinesterase inhibitor therapy.[50] The initiation of these therapies among hospice-eligible patients requires a thoughtful discussion that weighs the goals of care against the likely limited ability of these therapies to stabilize or prevent decline of a person's remaining cognitive and functional abilities. Clinicians often question the impact of discontinuing cholinesterase inhibitors in people with end-stage dementia. Although studies of patients with mild to moderate AD found that discontinuing cholinesterase inhibitor therapy leads to a precipitous cognitive and functional decline to nontreatment levels, investigations have not examined the impact of drug discontinuation in those with advanced dementia.

Side effects of cholinesterase inhibitors vary substantially but tend to decrease in frequency over time and occur less in people with advanced dementia. Gastrointestinal side effects including nausea, vomiting, and diarrhea are most common. Nausea occurs in less than 10% of patients who use donepezil but in almost 20% of patients using galantamine and 50% of patients using rivastigmine (oral formulation).[39,40,51,52] Vomiting is infrequent with donepezil and galantamine but occurs in more than 25% of patients who take rivastigmine (oral formulation). Diarrhea may occur with all three agents, although it is reported in fewer than 10% of cases. Weight loss is reported with rivastigmine and galantamine, averaging 2 kg overall. Stopping these medications in patients with advanced dementia may improve their appetite and weight. Dizziness is not uncommon but is reported more frequently with rivastigmine. Other less frequest side effects include muscle cramps, abnormal dreams (donepezil), syncope, gastrointestinal bleeding, and urinary incontinence.

Overall, cholinesterase inhibitor therapy has been consistently found to improve cognitive, functional, and behavioral outcomes in people with mild to moderate and moderate to severe AD. Studies in vascular dementia, Lewy body dementia, and PD-related dementia also show some benefit of cholinesterase inhibitor therapy compared with placebo, albeit the effect size tends to be lower.[52-54] Despite this proven benefit, some experts believe that cholinesterase inhibitors do not modify the underlying neurodegenerative process, that clinical differences between active therapy and placebo are statistically significant but clinically irrelevant, and that the financial cost (about $150 monthly for brand name drugs, which may decrease in cost as generics become more available) and side effects do not justify their ubiquitous use. To support this claim, opponents of cholinesterase inhibitors often cite the AD2000 study, a nationwide study conducted in England that was designed to assess the clinical relevance of donepezil therapy. The authors concluded that donepezil was not cost effective and that its benefits were below minimally relevant thresholds.[55] Unfortunately, the applicability of AD2000 study findings are limited because of the study's low participant enrollment; that is, the power calculation estimated that 3,000 participants would need to be enrolled to test the hypothesis that active drug therapy decreases primary outcomes of institutionalization, progress of disability, or the related cost-effectiveness measure. Only 566 (19% of target) participants were recruited into the trial; 76% of them were from a select region of the country.

Glutamate is an excitatory amino acid found in the brain, and with pathological conditions such as AD there is excessive stimulation of NMDA receptors by glutamate.[56] This overactivation is thought to play a role in AD-related cognitive impairments. Blockage of the NMDA receptor by memantine is thought to modulate, in a voltage-dependent manner, the passage of calcium through the ion channels associated with these receptors. It is believed that memantine prevents the neurotoxicity associated with NMDA receptor overactivation while allowing normal glutamine transmission in the brain.[57]

Two pivotal trials led the FDA to approve memantine for the treatment of moderate to severe AD (MMSE scores, 3-14).[58,59] These trials established the efficacy and safety of memantine monotherapy and combination therapy for patients already taking donepezil. Patients who received active treatment experienced improvement in cognition, functioning, behavior, and global impression of change. Memantine therapy was associated with significantly less deterioration than placebo on the SIB; the mean difference between groups was 6 points ($P < .001$). However, no difference in response was exhibited between memantine therapy and placebo on the neuropsychiatric inventory. Frequency of adverse events was similar in the active treatment and placebo groups, and there was no difference between memantine and placebo in the frequency of side effects.

The addition of memantine administration for patients with moderate to severe AD who already were taking donepezil resulted in additional patient and caregiver benefits compared with patients continuing on donepezil monotherapy. Statistically significant benefits of active treatment compared with placebo emerged by 4 weeks and persisted over the duration of the study to 24 weeks for both primary outcome measures. As in the previous study, rates of occurrence of adverse events in active treatment and placebo were similar between the two groups, and no difference in frequency of side effects existed between memantine and placebo. In addition, caregivers spent 45.8 fewer hours per month on average caring for patients in the memantine-treated group compared with the placebo group. Moreover, the dropout rate for both studies was higher in the placebo group than in the active treatment arm.

Memantine also has been studied in people with mild to moderate (MMSE scores, 10-24) Lewy body dementia and PD dementia.[60] Compared with placebo, the active treatment group of memantine, 20 mg daily, showed statistically significant improvements in clinical global impression of change and neuropsychiatric behaviors in people with Lewy body dementia but not PD dementia. However, in most of the cognitive testing and functional outcomes, no significant differences emerged between active treatment and placebo with either dementia group. The benefits observed with memantine were mild, with unclear clinical significance. Whether or not memantine is effective in more advanced stages of Lewy body dementia and PD dementia remains unknown.

Nonpharmacologic

An array of studies testing the benefits of nonpharmacologic therapies on cognitive, functional, and behavioral outcomes for people with dementia continue to be published. Studies to date generally focus on cognitive training, social engagement, and physical health and functioning. In addition to using these measures, healthcare providers should be aware of community resources and support services so they can refer people with dementia and their caregivers to available resources.

Cognitive training appears to be more useful for people with dementia when interventions target global cognitive status rather than specific cognitive domains.[61] Moreover, benefits have been found to increase when cognitive stimulation is combined with cholinesterase inhibitor therapy. One study that targeted specific cognitive domains found some improvements in functioning on select tasks, such as recall of personal information or face-name recall with a cognitive intervention, but the minor improvements noted did not generalize to neuropsychological measures (ie, verbal memory, visual memory, motor speed).[62] Although no approach can prevent cognitive deterioration over a prolonged period of time (eg, 2 years), no treatment is associated with greater and faster deterioration than any other treatment. Another approach being examined reviews patients' neuropsychological profiles and tailors interventions to emphasize an individual's strengths and mediate their weaknesses.

Investigations examining the role of social engagement found that disengagement was associated with an increased risk of cognitive decline.[63] During a 12-year period, older adults with the highest levels of social engagement were 30% less likely to experience a decline in dementia from none to mild, from mild to moderate, or from moderate to severe. Finally, intervention trials designed to foster social and intellectual engagement have helped enhance cognition in subjects with dementia over a short period, but whether these interventions lead to sustainable improvement in cognition and decreased the risk of institutionalization remains to be elucidated.[64]

Neurodegenerative diseases result in impaired mobility and functional decline. Multiple studies have found that exercise is associated with improved flexibility, balance, and strength among community-dwelling older adults and frail nursing home residents. One study conducted a 12-session, combined home exercise and behavioral management intervention involving patients with AD and their caregivers. At 3 months it was found that intervention-group patients exercised more often and had fewer days of restricted activity than control-group patients.[65] At 2 years intervention-group patients continued to have significantly better physical functioning scores. The intervention group also experienced the additional benefit of significantly lower depression scores than the control arm throughout the 2 years of the study. The study's authors concluded the intervention resulted in improved physical and emotional health of the patients with AD. A 2011 systematic review of the effects of physical activity on physical functioning, QOL, and depression found that physical activity interventions improve physical functioning in those with dementia.[66] However, evidence remains unclear as to whether these interventions decrease depression and improve QOL.

CLINICAL SITUATION CONTINUED FROM P. 5

Margaret's Case Continues

Margaret is diagnosed with moderate-stage dementia, most likely of the Alzheimer's type. Her physician starts her on cholinesterase inhibitor therapy, donepezil, 5 mg daily, to minimize side effects, with a plan to increase to the therapeutic dose of 10 mg daily after 4 weeks. Robert has taken a leave of absence from work to live with his mother while he decides how to best care for her. He now is managing her finances, cooking for her, driving her, and supervising her medication. On follow-up visits it is observed that her irritability has improved on the new medication.

Question Four

Robert is weary after assuming his increasing care burden but glad his mother is improving. He is trying to make arrangements for her care that will allow him to get back to work. He asks, "How long is this going to last? Will Mom have to go to a nursing home?" The *least* helpful response might be

A. "Have you talked with the social worker about available resources?"

B. "Patients who get good care can generally manage in their own homes."

C. "Your mother will need more help as time goes on, but when is hard to predict."

D. "Have you talked with your mother and other family members about care arrangements when Margaret needs more assistance?"

Correct Response and Analysis

B is the correct response. Supporting Robert is perhaps the most crucial thing that can be done to help Margaret now. Although each of the above statements may be true, the implication of B is that if Robert does a good job he can keep Margaret out of a nursing home. This is more guilt producing than helpful. Helping Robert communicate with his family about options, obtain resources, and make sensible plans is much more useful.

Question Five

What is the typical disease progression in persons with AD?

A. Rapid decline in cognitive and functional abilities

B. Slow progressive deterioration

C. Slow progressive deterioration punctuated by episodes of substantial cognitive and functional decline

D. Comorbidities and not AD by itself contribute to cognitive and functional decline.

Correct Response and Analysis

The correct response is C. Typically, AD has a protracted course with an average life expectancy of 4 to 7 years after diagnosis. The disease course is characterized by gradual cognitive and functional decline with episodes of substantive progression, usually in response to an acute illness. Rapid deterioration is not characteristic of AD. Although comorbidities frequently exist in people with AD and may facilitate cognitive and functional decline, other medical conditions by themselves have not been shown to be the primary impetus for cognitive and functional deterioration.

Question Six

What are the FDA-approved therapies for the treatment of moderate to severe AD?

A. Donepezil

B. Rivastigmine

C. Galantamine

D. Memantine

Correct Response and Analysis

The correct responses are A and D. Donepezil is the only cholinesterase inhibitor approved for the treatment of mild to moderate and moderate to severe AD. Memantine is the only NMDA receptor antagonist approved for the treatment of moderate to severe AD. Rivastigmine and galantamine are cholinesterase inhibitors approved for the treatment of mild to moderate AD.

Question Seven

What outcomes have been found to improve with cholinesterase therapy?

A. Global impression of change

B. Cognition

C. Function

D. Neuropsychiatric symptoms

Correct Response and Analysis

All of the responses above are correct. In people with mild to moderate AD, cholinesterase inhibitor therapy has been found to improve or ameliorate cognitive, functional, and behavioral domains compared with placebo. Active treatment with a cholinesterase inhibitor also is associated with demonstrable benefits in global impression of change based on caregiver report and clinical observation.

Question Eight

What additional pharmacologic therapy may benefit this patient?

A. Antipsychotic

B. Antidepressant

C. NMDA receptor antagonist

D. A second cholinesterase inhibitor

Correct Response and Analysis

The correct response is C. The NMDA receptor antagonist memantine, along with cholinesterase inhibitors, has been shown to provide cognitive, functional, and behavioral benefits compared with placebo in people with moderate-stage AD. Compared with donepezil monotherapy, combination therapy with donepezil and memantine has been associated with superior cognitive, functional, and behavioral outcomes. Data are not available to guide which therapy—a cholinesterase inhibitor or NMDA receptor antagonist—should be initiated first. A second cholinesterase inhibitor should not be added. Margaret's irritability has improved, suggesting that an antipsychotic is not indicated. Also, she has not displayed signs and symptoms of depression to warrant a trial of an antidepressant.

Question Nine

What are the most common side effects of cholinesterase inhibitors?

A. Nausea

B. Sleepiness

C. Vomiting

D. Diarrhea

Correct Response and Analysis

The correct responses are A, C, and D. The most frequent side effects of cholinesterase inhibitors are gastrointestinal nausea, vomiting, poor appetite, and diarrhea. Dizziness is also a frequent adverse effect of cholinesterase-inhibitor therapy. Cholinesterase inhibitors have not been associated with increased sleepiness.

Continued on page 23

Life Expectancies After Diagnosis

Prognostication

Prognosis in dementia, both at the time of diagnosis and after a person reaches the advanced stage, is an area of much debate and research. Initial studies examining life expectancy for people with dementia suggested median survival is approximately 10 years.[67] However, these studies were limited to including patients into the study at the time of entry instead of at the time of diagnosis, a circumstance that introduced a selection bias. Studies conducted between 1990 and 2010 that ascertain survival at time of diagnosis suggest a much shorter life expectancy, with a mean survival of 4 to 7 years.[22-24] Variables associated with shorter survival in these studies included older age at onset, male gender, gait disturbance, wandering, comorbid medical conditions (particularly diabetes, cerebrovascular disease, and cardiovascular disease), a history of falls, and extrapyramidal signs. Survival was not associated with ethnicity, education, behavioral disturbances, dementia diagnosis, or symptoms of depression.

Determining life expectancy is particularly challenging near EOL and can limit patients' access to hospice enrollment.[68,69] Hospice criteria currently in use for dementia do a poor job of predicting 6-month mortality and exhibit the greatest variability in survival among all hospice diagnoses (**Table 3**).[70-72] In an effort to improve prediction of 6-month mortality, two risk score models have been developed using nursing home data from the Minimum Data Set (MDS): the Mortality Risk Index (MRI) and Advanced Dementia Prognostic Tool (ADEPT). The MRI

Table 3. Primary Factors for Predicting 6-Month Mortality in Dementia: National Hospice and Palliative Care Organization Guideline for Certification of Hospice Eligibility

Severity of dementia ≥ FAST stage 7-C
- Inability to walk, dress, or bathe without assistance
- Urinary and fecal incontinence
- Inability to speak more than six different intelligible words per day

Severe comorbid condition within past 6 months
- Aspiration pneumonia
- Pyelonephritis
- Septicemia
- Multiple, progressive stage 3 to 4 decubiti
- Fever after antibiotics

Inability to maintain fluid/caloric intake to sustain life if feeding tube is in place
- Weight loss > 10% in 6 months
- Serum albumin < 2.5 g/dL

Note. NHPCO recommends that providers research the local coverage determinations (LCDs) that apply to their state by using the Medicare coverage database, which can be found at www.cms.gov/medicare-coverage-database/overview-and-quick-search. aspx (Accessed February 6, 2012). These LCDs will provide information regarding disease-specific factors and prognosis, because the final determination and information about disease appropriateness rests with each hospice Medicare Administrative Contractor (MAC). We include this information here as a starting point for determining a patient's eligibility for hospice services but encourage physicians to refer to their LCDs and MACs for current information (NHPCO, personal communication, January 27, 2012). Summarized from NHPCO's Medical Guidelines for Determining Prognosis in Selected Non-Cancer Diseases, 2nd ed. © 1997 National Hospice Organization. Adapted with permission. All rights reserved.[77]

---

retrospectively examined potential variables for which 12 characteristics were identified as predictive of 6-month survival using a derivation and validation cohort (**Table 4**).[73] The authors also compared the effectiveness of their tool with the functional component of the hospice criteria. The risk score demonstrated better discrimination to predict 6-month mortality; however, the risk tool was not compared with the actual hospice criteria, which require specific functional limitations and the presence of disease complications (eg, aspiration pneumonia, upper urinary-tract infection, septicemia, multiple decubitus ulcers [stage 3 or 4], recurrent fever despite antibiotics, or inability to take in fluids or food to sustain life).[74] Other limitations of the MRI include the reliance on retrospective data, only two states being represented, and the inclusion of only recent nursing home admissions.

The ADEPT tool was an attempt to overcome the limitations of the MRI by prospectively collecting MDS data to develop and validate a prognostic measure while simultaneously gathering clinical information related to hospice eligibility criteria.[75] The following variables were most predictive of 6-month mortality: nursing home stay less than 90 days, increasing age, male gender, shortness of breath, one or more pressure sores at stage 2 or above, complete functional dependence, bedfast most of day, insufficient oral intake, bowel incontinence, body mass index (BMI) lower than 18.5, recent weight loss, and congestive heart failure (CHF). Risk points were ascribed for each condition based upon the strength of association with 6-month mortality. Risk score ranges were generated and mortality rates within each range calculated. The ADEPT model only performed slightly better than traditional hospice criteria, with an area under the receiver operating characteristic curve of 0.58 versus 0.55, respectively. As with the MRI, the ADEPT was based on nursing home patients and did not incorporate the degree of caregiver support or willingness to pursue interventions such as hospitalization, administration of antibiotics or intravenous (IV) fluids, dialysis, or enteral nutrition, which may impact survival.[76]

Overall, efforts to more accurately predict survival among patients with dementia near EOL have not improved significantly or resulted in newer models, reinforcing the importance of focusing efforts on better delineation of goals of care that reflect a patient's clinical status and previously expressed wishes. It is hoped that hospice, the current reimbursement structure for state-of-the-art EOL care, will consider adopting this focused approach for enrollment because it is more reflective of clinical practice.

Communication and Hope

Dementia is a progressive illness that gradually robs a person of the ability to communicate. For patients with advanced dementia, nonverbal communication may continue to provide useful information about their symptoms, unmet needs, and experiences up to the time of death.

Table 4. Characteristics Associated with 6-Month Mortality Among Nursing Home Residents with Advanced Dementia	
Characteristic	Mortality Risk (%)*
Complete functional dependence	1.9
Male gender	1.9
Cancer diagnosis	1.7
Oxygen requirement	1.6
Congestive heart failure	1.6
Shortness of breath	1.5
Less than 25% of food consumed	1.5
Unstable medical condition	1.5
Bowel incontinence	1.5
Bedfast	1.5
Older than 83 years	1.4
Not awake most of the morning and afternoon	1.4

* Based on the hazard ratio using a stepwise multivariate Cox proportional hazards model.

Healthcare providers are called to continue to identify individuals with progressive dementia as a whole person with a spiritual, emotional, social, and physical presence. Through ongoing connection with the family and patient, healthcare providers can continue to offer hope and meaning to their respective experiences and roles.

Symptom Control

Pain

Evaluating the pain experience of a person with dementia can be challenging because of the person's short-term memory impairment and decrements in language and executive functioning. Although cortical processing of pain impulses may be altered, pain pathways in the peripheral and central nervous systems usually are spared from underlying neurodegenerative changes. That is, parenchymal brain changes that lead to cognitive impairment may modify the perception of pain by altering signal processing within the amygdala, thereby decreasing the affective contribution of pain, which in turn lessens reported pain intensity. Despite this theoretical concern, laboratory studies demonstrate that those with mild to moderate cognitive impairment maintain pain thresholds similar to those of cognitively intact populations.[78]

Given that dementia predominately is a disease of older adults and that a large percentage of older adults have chronic medical conditions associated with acute or persistent pain, it is not surprising that pain is such a pervasive symptom among persons with dementia. Cross-sectional studies report a prevalence of pain between 50% and 85% in ambulatory and long-term care settings, respectively.[79-83] Moreover, compared with cognitively intact control groups, patients with cognitive impairment are at higher risk for receiving inadequate analgesia.[84] Arthritis is the second most common chronic condition in all older adults (reported behind hypertension), with 50% of people older than 65 years reporting an arthritis diagnosis and 46% citing chronic joint symptoms.[85] Compounding the problem is that multiple rather than single joint involvement is typical in the older adult population. A 2006 study found that, on average, subjects reported four joints causing pain or stiffness most of the time during the previous 3 months.[86] In addition, many conditions associated with acute pain in older adults, such as postherpetic neuralgia and postfracture pain, lead to persistent pain. See **Table 5** for common conditions associated with noncancer pain in older adults.

A thorough pain assessment for patients with dementia includes patient self-report, caregiver report, and direct observation of pain behaviors.[79,87] Pain is a subjective experience that has no objective test, and self-report is the benchmark.[79] Research continues to corroborate data that pain self-report scales demonstrate concurrent validity and reliability in cognitively intact and mildly to moderately impaired patient populations.[80] When asking patients about pain, clinicians should direct questions to the present

Table 5. Common Conditions Associated with Noncancer Pain in Older Adults

Condition	Increases in Prevalence with Age
Osteoarthritis	Yes
Crystal arthropathy (gout and pseudogout)	Yes
Osteoporosis	Yes
Claudication	Yes
Postherpetic neuralgia	Yes
Spinal stenosis	Yes
Fibromyalgia	Yes
Diabetic peripheral neuropathy	Probably
Constipation	Yes
Fractures	Yes

pain they experience at rest and with activity. As dementia progresses to a more advanced stage, clinicians should continue to ask verbal patients about their present pain experience. At the same time, to ascertain whether a nonverbal patient is experiencing pain, healthcare providers need to incorporate the caregiver's report into their assessment as well as any nonverbal pain indicators from the patient.

Observing patients at rest and during activity provides another method to ascertain the pain experience. As dementia progresses to an advanced stage and patients experience substantial memory impairment and language deficits, nonverbal pain indicators become an important assessment tool.[88] A comprehensive webite summarizing some of the most commonly used measures with information on validity and reliability can be accessed at http://prc.coh.org/PAIN-NOA.htm. Consensus recommendations among an expert group supported the use of the Pain Assessment in Advanced Dementia (PAINAD) and Pain Assessment Checklist for Seniors with Limited Ability to Communicate (PACSLAC) to assess pain in nonverbal nursing home residents.[89] In fact, the group recommended each scale be used to screen for pain behaviors along with direct observation for other common pain behaviors. The PAINAD includes measures of breathing, negative vocalizations, facial expressions, body language, and consolability. The PACSLAC is organized into behaviors that fall into four groups: facial expressions, activity/body movement, social/personality/mood indicators, and physiologic indicators/sleeping changes/eating/vocal behaviors. Other tools, such as the Checklist of Nonverbal Pain Indicators (CNPI), have not been as extensively validated in persistent pain but maintain good face validity and are easy to use in clinical practice.[90] The CNPI behaviors include nonverbal vocalizations (ie, sighs, gasps, moans, groans, cries), facial grimacing and wincing (ie, furrowed brow, clenched teeth, tightening lips), bracing (ie, holding onto affected area at rest or during movement), rubbing, restlessness (ie, shifting position or inability to keep still), and vocal complaints. Some behaviors included in these scales lack specificity and may be the result of other symptoms or part of the underlying neurodegenerative process.[91] As a result, experts in pain and dementia suggest that if pain is on the differential diagnosis for the observed behavior, an empirical analgesic trial may be indicated.[79,87] With such an approach, an analgesic is prescribed for a specific behavior. Pain is considered a contributor to the behavior if its frequency or severity lessens or if it subsides altogether with analgesia.[92]

Another consideration in pain management is a patient's pain signature.[87] Because pain is a unique and multidimensional experience for each person, patients frequently develop a particular individualized response whenever they experience pain. For instance, a patient in pain may stop eating, refrain from social activities, become agitated, wander, or develop insomnia. In such cases, an analgesic trial may be appropriate to determine whether the patient's change in condition is the result of untreated or undertreated pain.

Caregivers can provide a more extensive history of a patient's pain experience, especially as short-term memory worsens. As described in the cancer literature, caregivers of those with mild to moderate dementia report patients have more pain than they indicate in their self-reports. Caregivers rarely overlook significant pain in patients.[81] At the same time, caregivers can provide valuable information about whether patients are taking prescribed analgesics, and they can describe any side effects.

Professional organizations and experts in the field recommend following the World Health

Organization (WHO) guidelines for cancer pain for the treatment of noncancer pain.[79] Although some controversy exists concerning the use of opioids for noncancer pain in healthier people, those with advanced illness who experience pain should not be denied safe and effective therapy. Opioids can safely and effectively be used to treat suspected pain, even for people with advanced dementia.[93] Many clinicians hesitate to use opioids for patients with dementia for fear their confusion may worsen or they may develop delirium. However, a review article on the cognitive effects of opioids suggests these fears are exaggerated.[94] In fact, evidence suggests opioid use may decrease delirium in some populations.[95] See *UNIPAC 3* for more information on pain management.

Behavioral and Psychological Symptoms in Dementia

Even though behavioral and psychological symptoms in dementia (BPSD) are not currently included in the diagnostic criteria for AD, non-cognitive symptoms represent an important and frequently overlooked aspect of AD care. BPSDs include apathy, affective syndrome (ie, anxiety, depression), psychomotor (ie, agitation, irritability, and aberrant motor) behavior, psychosis (ie, delusions and hallucinations), and mania (ie, dishinhibition and euphoria); all except affective syndrome show an increase in severity with disease progression.[96,97] In addition to their impact on patients, BPSDs are associated with depression and greater burden for caregivers as well as a higher incidence of institutionalization of those with dementia.[98]

Mood Disorders

Depression frequently occurs in people with dementia. For mild to moderate dementia, several standardized instruments—including the 30-item Geriatric Depression Scale, the Brief Carroll Depression Rating Scale, and the Cornell Depression Rating Scale—have been validated.[99-101] For people with moderate to severe dementia, self-report measures are less reliable and valid. Clinicians should consider evaluating for depression if patients experience changes in mood, behavior, cognition, functioning, sleep, or appetite; weight loss; social withdrawal; or apathy. Given the wide variability in the expression of depression in people with advanced dementia and the limited ability of these patients to verbally communicate their experience, an empiric trial of an antidepressant for several weeks may be indicated.

Few studies exist that describe the natural history of depression in dementia. One study that followed patients with mild to moderate dementia monthly for 1 year revealed an annual incidence of 10.6% for major depression and 29.8% for minor depression. Persistent depression lasting 6 months or longer occurred in 20% of patients.[102] Prevalence rates vary widely depending on study population and referral patterns, with major depression affecting 20% to 25% of people with dementia and an additional 20% to 30% of those with minor symptoms.[103,104] In addition to being common, the assessment and management of depression is important because depression negatively influences self-perceived QOL.[105]

Both nonpharmacologic and pharmacologic therapies are appropriate treatment options for depression in those with dementia, but to date few studies have been conducted in either area.

Pharmacologic therapy is usually based on the neuropathological changes associated with depression in patients with Alzheimer's dementia; in particular, loss of noradrenergic cells in the locus coeruleus and serotonergic raphe nuclei.[106] Selective serotonin reuptake inhibitors (SSRIs) are considered first-line therapy by some experts because they have the most data supporting efficacy; however, dosages may need to be increased to obtain optimal effect.[107,108] The tricyclic antidepressent nortriptyline also resulted in clinically significant improvement compared with placebo, but, because of side effects, 34% of participants randomized to active drug therapy had the drug discontinued.[109] Newer agents that maintain dual inhibition of the norepinephrine and serotonin systems have not been studied. One study found the stimulant methylphenidate improved depressive symptoms in dementia. However, clinicians must monitor for psychosis, which can frequently begin or worsen when methylphenidate therapy is initiated in people with dementia.[110,111] Nonpharmacologic therapies that have been successful in decreasing depressive symptoms include cognitive, music, and recreational therapies.[112] Research has not examined the theoretical benefit of combining nonpharmacologic and pharmacologic therapies. A small study has suggested significant clinical benefits with the use of electroconvulsive therapy to manage refractory depression, although people with dementia were significantly more likely to have cognitive decline after 6 months of treatment compared with those without dementia.[113] See *UNIPAC 2* for a general approach to the treatment of depression in those with dementia.

Apathy

Apathy frequently is confused with depression. It is a common symptom of AD and other neurodegenerative conditions, with a prevalence higher than 50%.[114] Moreover, it occurs early in the disease course and can persist. Apathy can be defined as a loss of motivation and manifests as diminished initiation, lowered interest, decreasing social engagement, blunted emotions, and lack of insight.[115] Apathy differs from depression in that no symptoms of altered mood are present. Differentiation is important because antidepressants have a minimal effect in the treatment of apathy, but psychostimulants and cholinergic therapy may be of some benefit.[111,115,116]

Psychosis

Psychotic symptoms in dementia consist of delusions and hallucinations. Studies conducted between 2002 and 2006 of psychotic symptoms in dementia suggest a point prevalence of delusions between 18% and 35%, whereas hallucinations are reported in 10% to 20% of patients.[117-119] Visual hallucinations are part of the core diagnostic criteria for Lewy body dementia and occur in as many as 77% of patients.[120] Risk factors for developing psychosis include severity of dementia, African-American ethnicity, extrapyramidal symptoms, and sensory impairment.[121,122]

Numerous RCTs and a meta-analysis suggest modest efficacy of antipsychotics over placebo in the treatment of delusions and hallucinations and no apparent efficacy advantage between typical and atypical antipsychotics.[123-125] Antipsychotic selection is based on practical considerations such as route of administration and side effect profile. For example, quetiapine frequently is the drug of choice in patients with parkinsonian symptoms, olanzapine as a dissolvable wafer can be placed on the tongue for patients who cannot swallow pills, and risperidone liquid can be administered through feeding tubes. **Table 6** lists frequently used atypical antipsychotics and recommended dosages. However, side effects are a notable downside and are perceived to be more numerous with typical antipsychotics. A large randomized trial found increased costs with no improvement in QOL and functional outcomes associated with second-generation antipsychotics for patients with AD and psychosis.[126]

Treatment for delusions and hallucinations with antipsychotics must be carefully considered. This is particularly true for patients with Lewy body dementia, for whom antipsychotics have been associated with marked worsening

Table 6. Atypical Antipsychotic Use for Dementia*

Antipsychotic	Recommended Dosage	Available Formulations	Frequency	Remarkable Characteristics
Risperidone	0.25 mg-2.0 mg/d	Tablet	Twice daily	Extrapyramidal symptoms; dose dependent
		Disintegrating tablet		
		Liquid		
		Intramuscular injection		
Olanzapine	2.5 mg-15 mg/d	Tablet	Once or twice daily	Weight gain and hyperglycemia more common
		Disintegrating tablet		
Quetiapine	25 mg-400 mg/d	Immediate- or extended-release tablet	Two or three times daily	Fewer extrapyramidal effects; most sedating
Aripiprazole	5 mg-30 mg/d	Tablet	Once or twice daily	Less likely to prolong QT interval
		Disintegrating tablet		
		Liquid		

Atypical antipsychotics listed in this table are associated with QT prolongation, weight gain, hyperglycemia, stroke, and death. Newer atypical antipsychotics are not recommended because of the lack of RCTs in elderly people with dementia.

Editors' note. The US Food and Drug Administration (FDA) added black box warnings to several medications commonly used by hospice and palliative care practitioners. Black box warnings are designed to highlight the potential for rare but serious medical complications such as stroke or myocardial infarction associated with the use of these drugs. Hospice and palliative care practitioners should be aware of these FDA black box warnings and the risk-benefit ratio of these medications and alternatives for individual patients. The short prognosis and critical importance of symptom relief for many hospice and palliative care patients may justify the use of these medications despite such risks.

of rigidity, locked-in syndrome, and even death. For patients with Lewy body dementia and their caregivers, for whom psychosis is particularly bothersome, a trial of the antipsychotic quetiapine (which is considered to cause fewer of these side effects than other antipsychotics) or any of the cholinesterase inhibitors may be indicated. Patients and their caregivers should be assured that these symptoms frequently occur in neurodegenerative diseases, and, if the symptoms are not bothersome to them, pharmacologic therapy likely poses greater risk than close clinical follow-up.[127] Class-related side effects of atypical antipsychotics include weight gain (most concerning with olanzapine), metabolic abnormalities (eg, dyslipidemia, glucose intolerance), QT prolongation, and cerebrovascular events. In a pooled analysis of 3,353 patients on atypical antipsychotics and 1,757 on placebo, active treatment was associated with an increased risk of death (3.5% vs 2.3%, respectively; odds ratio,

1.54 [1.06-2.23]; P = .02; risk difference 0.01 [.004-.02]; P = .01).[128] Stated another way, for every 100 people treated with an antipsychotic, 9 to 25 persons will be helped, there would be one or two cerebrovascular events, and one death. Antipsychotics carry an FDA black box warning for increased risk of strokes and death in patients with dementia. Additional common side effects of typical and atypical antipsychotics include sedation, extra-pyramidal effects, edema, and infections.

General principles should be considered before initiating pharmacologic management of psychosis and agitation with antipsychotics. The first step is to try and identify potential contributors to the symptom (eg, anticholinergic medication leading to hallucinations). Next, a thoughtful discussion regarding overall risks and benefits and other treatment options should take place. Identify the target symptom and evaluate other therapies' effectiveness at a specified time point (generally 2-4 weeks). It also is important to use the lowest dosage of medication possible to achieve clinical effectiveness, so start low and go slow. Monitor effectiveness and, if the target symptom abates, strongly consider decreasing the medication dose or stopping it altogether. Finally, as with any medication, monitor safety by frequently assessing for side effects. As with any symptomatic therapy, treatment needs to be considered in the context of how bothersome the symptoms are for the patient or caregiver, the goals of care, and the potential benefits compared to risks of the therapy. Consultation with a geriatric psychiatrist may be warranted.

Agitation

Many definitions of the term *agitation* exist and each has relative strengths and weaknesses. Recent studies have indicated the prevalence of agitation throughout a 1-month period among patients with dementia is between 36% and 52%.[117-119] One difficulty with this term is it is imprecise and can be applied to a variety of conditions such as delirium, depression, terminal symptoms, or a manifestation of the underlying dementia itself. The term does not help distinguish among potential contributing causes that have been established in the literature, including physical symptoms (eg, pain, sleep disturbances), psychological symptoms (eg, depression), medical illness (eg, delirium, seizure disorder, constipation, urinary retention), unmet needs (eg, hunger, social isolation, soiled diaper), environment (eg, unfamiliar surroundings causing fear, overstimulation or understimulation), medications (eg, theophylline, caffeine, digoxin), and the underlying neurodegenerative process itself (**Table 7**).[129] Also, agitation must be differentiated from resistance to care, which requires a different management approach. To help differentiate from among the multitude of potential contributors to agitation, healthcare providers should ascertain the context in which the behavior occurs. Finally, the nonspecificity of the term may result in a single-treatment approach with medications that have substantial side effects.[130] As with other BPSDs, agitation has been associated with caregiver depression and poor mental and physical health.[131]

Many standardized scales exist to measure behavioral disturbances. One of the most widely used scales is the Cohen-Mansfield Agitation Inventory. The instrument was constructed and tested for validity among nursing home residents and has since been validated in other settings.[132] Factor analysis revealed three categories: (a) aggressive behavior (verbal aggression such as screaming and cursing or physical aggression such as hitting and scratching), (b) physical nonaggressive behavior (pacing, hiding things, restlessness, wandering), and (c) verbal nonaggressive behaviors (repeated requests for attention, complaining, interrupting).[133] In studies of people with dementia that use this scale, aggressive behaviors are more commonly found in men, specifically those with a premorbid history of aggression, greater cognitive impairment, and conflict with their caregiver.[134] Physical nonaggressive behaviors are associated with better physical health and greater cognitive impairment.[135] Verbal agitation is associated with female gender, social isolation, sensory impairment, pain, physical restraints, and functional impairment.[136]

Depending on the contributing etiologies of agitation, pharmacologic and nonpharmacologic treatment approaches should be considered. Nonpharmacologic interventions can be divided into three broad categories[137]:
- unmet needs intervention—conceptualizes the behavior as an underlying need
- learning and behavioral intervention—behavior leads to a consequence that reinforces continuation of the undesirable behavior

Table 7. Causes Contributing to Agitation in Dementia

Contributing Cause	Consideration	Treatment Approach
Physical symptom	Pain	Analgesics
	Sleep disturbance	Behavior modification, sedative-hypnotic drugs
Psychological symptom	Depression	Antidepressant
Medical illness	Delirium	Evaluate predisposing causes
	Seizure disorder	Treat underlying condition
	Constipation	
	Urinary retention	
	Psychosis	
	Dehydration	
	Infection	
Unmet need	Hunger	Attend to need
	Social isolation	
	Soiled diaper	
Sensory impairment	Vision loss	Adaptive devices
	Hearing loss	
Environment	Unfamiliar surroundings	Modify environment
	Overstimulation	
	Understimulation	
Medication/substance	Digoxin	Decrease dosage or discontinue agent
	Theophylline	
	Methyphenidate	
	Caffeine	
	Antipsychotic	
	Benzodiazepine	
Underlying dementia	Alzheimer's disease	Evaluate severity of symptom and consider risk-benefit ratio of available treatments
	Vascular dementia	
	Lewy body dementia	
	Mixed dementia	
	Other	

- environmental vulnerability and reduced stress thresholds intervention—a mismatch between the setting and the patient's ability to deal with it.

In a recent meta-analysis, the study's authors concluded that nonpharmacologic interventions that address unmet needs and behavioral issues can be efficacious. Because of the relationship between unmet needs and agitation, changes in behavior should prompt screening for elder mistreatment.[137]

Since the publication of the meta-analysis, several promising well-conducted nonpharmacologic treatment strategies have emerged as being helpful for agitation in people with dementia. A couple of small RCTs have demonstrated significant benefits in decreasing agitation with aromatherapy.[129] A family caregiver intervention of community-dwelling people with moderate dementia found substantial improvement in the most problematic behavior identified, including agitation; 67.5% improvement occurred in the intervention group versus 45.8% improvement in the no-treatment control ($P < .01$).[138] The intervention consisted of multiple home and telephone contacts performed by nurses and occupational therapists over 16 weeks, with the goal of identifying behavior triggers and training caregivers in strategies to modify the trigger and modify their reaction. Unfortunately, as with many nonpharmacologic interventions, the study's benefits appeared to wane over time. Lastly, a nursing home study implemented a patient-centered approach in which standard stimuli were introduced to people with moderate to severe dementia and agitation.[139] The stimuli included live social (a real baby, dog, and one-on-one socializing), task (flower arranging and coloring), reading, music listening, work (stamping envelopes, folding clothes, and sorting items), simulated social (a doll, plush animal, and robotic animal), manipulative (squeeze ball, activity pillow, building blocks, fabric book, wallet for men and purse for women, and puzzle), and usual care. The study demonstrated that any type of stimulus was preferable to standard nursing home care; the stimuli more effectively addressed physical agitation than verbal agitation, and live social stimuli generally was most effective.

Pharmacologic studies that examine the benefits of active drug therapy compared with placebo for the treatment of agitation fail to consider the numerous contributors to agitation and most often assume that a given symptom is related to the underlying neurodegenerative disease. Pharmacologic treatment should be considered only after a patient with dementia and his or her caregiver have undergone a thorough history to discern potential contributors to the agitation. This evaluation should be followed by a focused physical examination and relevant laboratory or radiologic studies. When the clinician is confident the agitation is related to the underlying dementia, the pharmacologic treatments described in this book may be considered.

As with treatment for psychosis and delusions, evidence suggests typical and atypical antipsychotics are modestly effective as agitation treatment for people with dementia, but they can cause significant side effects.[123-125] Additional agents that have been used for the treatment of agitation for dementia are displayed in **Table 8** and include antidepressants such as trazodone and SSRIs,[140-142] cholinesterase inhibitors,[42] NMDA receptor antagonists,[143] anxiolytics (ie, benzodiazepines),[144] and anticonvulsants such as valproate, carbamezapine, and gabapentin.[145-147] The literature on the effectiveness of these agents is mixed, and their use should be weighed carefully against relative efficacy, adverse effects, and cost.

Geriatric treatment principles are paramount when considering use of pharmacologic agents to treat agitation in dementia, especially because patients with dementia have diminished cognitive and functional reserves. After an appropriate evaluation and treatment of any contributing conditions, consider whether the agitation results in enough patient or caregiver distress to warrant treatment. If treatment is warranted, a nonpharmacologic approach should be considered first. If pharmacologic therapy is determined to be the appropriate next step, establish a clear treatment goal and consider discontinuing the medication if there is no discernable improvement within several weeks of therapy initiation. Considering the side-effect profile of currently available medications, begin with the lowest possible effective dosage and titrate upward slowly until the goal of therapy is achieved. Because BPSDs can change over time, consider lowering the dosage or discontinuing the therapy altogether to see whether the behavior recurs.

Table 8. Pharmacologic Approaches to Treatment of Agitation in Dementia

AGENT	DOSAGE (STARTING, MAXIMAL)	EVIDENCE	COMMON SIDE EFFECTS
Atypical antipsychotics*	See Table 6	RCT	See Table 6
Trazodone	25 mg-50 mg, 300 mg/d	RCT	Sedation, postural hypotension
SSRIs			
Citalopram	10 mg/d, 20 mg/d	RCT	Nausea, insomnia, somnolence
Anticonvulsants			
Carbamazepine	100 mg/d, 400 mg/d (100 mg 4 times/d)	RCT	Sedation, rash, anemia, hepatotoxicity
Valproic acid	125 mg/d, 1,000 mg/d	RCT	Sedation, nausea, hepatotoxicity
Benzodiazepines			
Lorazepam	0.25 mg twice daily, 4 mg/d	RCT	Ataxia, sedation, falls, "paradoxical" agitation
Cholinesterase inhibitors	See Table 2	RCT	See Table 2
NMDA receptor antagonists	See Table 2	RCT	See Table 2

RCT, randomized controlled trial.

*Editors' note. The US Food and Drug Administration (FDA) added black box warnings to several medications commonly used by hospice and palliative care practitioners. Black box warnings are designed to highlight the potential for rare but serious medical complications such as stroke or myocardial infarction associated with the use of these drugs. Hospice and palliative care practitioners should be aware of these FDA black box warnings and the risk-benefit ratio of these medications and alternatives for individual patients. The short prognosis and critical importance of symptom relief for many hospice and palliative care patients may justify the use of these medications despite such risks.

CLINICAL SITUATION CONTINUED FROM P. 13

Margaret's Case Continues

Four years after diagnosis Margaret is living in a nursing home. She is dependent in all of her IADLs, and although she is continent and can feed herself, she now requires assistance with bathing, dressing, and transferring. Two years ago memantine was added to her regimen because of a progressive decline in her cognition and functioning while on a cholinesterase inhibitor. Margaret recently developed aggressive behaviors, including screaming and hitting caregivers, and these behaviors have not responded to antidepressants and behavioral therapy. After risks and benefits were discussed with Robert, she was started on quetiapine, an antipsychotic drug, and her condition has been stable for 6 months. Margaret has presented to the physician's office with worsening aggression, agitation, and social withdrawal during the past 2 weeks. Because of the change in her behaviors, her quetiapine dose was increased.

Question Ten

Robert calls, extremely concerned about his mother's agitation. He says the nursing home has threatened to discharge his mother or send her to the hospital for evaluation because her behavior is so disruptive. She hit Robert when he was trying to help her dress. "Can't you give her a stronger tranquillizer?" he begs. Which of the following might be the best approach?

A. Arrange for ambulance transfer to the hospital for lumbar puncture and neurologic consultation.

B. Remind Robert of Margaret's resistance to nursing home care and suggest that Robert take Margaret back home.

C. Begin phenobarbital injections for palliative sedation.

D. Visit Margaret, examine her, and talk with her caregivers.

Correct Response and Analysis

D is the correct response. Although meningitis or missing home may be the cause of agitation in a few patients, it is highly unlikely that one of these is the issue now. Margaret is not close to death from her disease, and a less extreme measure than palliative sedation may be effective. A careful examination and discussion with her caregivers is certainly the best next step.

Question Eleven

What is the differential diagnosis of agitation and/or aggression in people with dementia?

A. A physical or psychological symptom

B. A concomitant medical illness

C. Change in environment

D. An underlying neurodegenerative process

Correct Response and Analysis

All of the above responses are correct. Assessment of agitation requires a broad and thoughtful approach. Only after a comprehensive evaluation can agitation and aggression be considered the result of the underlying neurodegenerative process. Potential contributors to agitation and aggression include physical symptoms, sensory impairment, psychological symptoms, medical illness, medications, unmet needs, and environment.

Question Twelve

What adverse effects are associated with the use of antipsychotic therapy in people with dementia?

A. Extrapyramidal effects

B. Hyperglycemia

C. QT prolongation

D. Stroke

Correct Response and Analysis

All of the answers listed are correct. Compared to typical antipsychotics, the newer atypical antipsychotics are thought to have fewer adverse effects. However, large randomized controlled clinical trials comparing atypical antipsychotic use with placebo for the treatment of agitation in persons with dementia have uncovered additional risks including stroke and death. These risks remain small and must be taken in context of the potential clinical benefits. Additional side effects reported with atypical antipsychotic use are weight gain, hyperglycemia, lipid dysregulation, and QT prolongation. Extrapyramidal effects can still occur with atypical antipsychotic use and may be medication and dosage related.

Question Thirteen

Which of the following statements are true regarding depression and apathy in people with dementia?

A. Depression and apathy frequently occur in people with dementia.

B. Apathy differs from depression in that it is not associated with a mood disturbance.

C. Depression and apathy readily respond to antidepressant therapy.

D. Depression and apathy can be associated with loss of interest.

Correct Response and Analysis

The correct answers are A, B, and D. Both apathy and depression frequently occur in people with dementia, but they are distinct clinical entities. Although both depression and apathy can be characterized by loss of interest, social disengagement, and emotional blunting, apathy differs because it is not associated with mood changes. Also, depression typically responds well to an antidepressant medication, but apathy generally is refractory to pharmacologic therapy.

The Case Continues

At the nursing home, Margaret is complaining of poor appetite and difficulty sleeping. Cognitively she is oriented to person and place, recalls zero out of three words at 5 minutes, and has intact attention. Her vital signs are normal, but she has lost 7 pounds since her last appointment 1 month ago. On physical examination her right knee is swollen and painful with decreased range of motion. There is no evidence of fecal impaction or urinary retention. Laboratory measurements, including urinalysis, were negative. An X ray of the knee revealed a moderate-sized effusion with chondrocalcinosis. Margaret was placed on a steroid taper with around-the-clock acetaminophen. Within a few days her pain decreased significantly, her appetite improved, she became more social, and her agitation resolved. This allowed the quetiapine dosage to be decreased to the previously prescribed level.

Continued on page 27

End-Stage Issues

As a dementia progresses to the advanced stage, the affected person becomes dependent upon others for all of his or her care. At the end stage, people with dementia are bed-bound, incontinent of stool and urine, develop difficulty handling secretions, and utter few if any intelligible words. This stage places patients at high risk for developing complications such as acute infection (urinary-tract infection, pneumonia), swallowing difficulties (dysphagia, aspiration), injuries and trauma (hip or other bone fractures), and stroke.[6,31,32,148] Ideally, before the patient develops an acute event, healthcare providers and the patient's power of attorney should discuss treatment preferences to consider once a complication develops. *UNIPAC 6* outlines ethical principles to consider (beneficence, autonomy, nonmaleficence, justice) when making treatment decisions for vulnerable patients with limited life expectancy and describes a framework for considering these complex issues.

Conversations with families about end-stage issues remain particularly important because patients dying of dementia often receive suboptimal EOL care that includes poor symptom control, inappropriate procedures, and placement in restraints.[149] At the same time, hospice is underused for people dying from dementia[76,150] even though multiple studies document its benefits for patients and families.[151-154]

The goal of this section is to provide healthcare professionals with the medical knowledge to conduct a thoughtful and accurate dialogue with surrogates to help them weigh the burdens and benefits associated with medical therapies commonly used near EOL.

Eating Difficulties

Dementia predisposes patients to eating and swallowing difficulties such as diminished reserve, apraxia, and dysphagia. Mealtime represents a stimulating experience that can overwhelm a person with dementia through visual, auditory, and olfactory sensory activation. When apraxia develops, a patient with dementia does not recognize food and forgets how to use utensils. Finger foods and large spoons can help. Also, cups should be small and not have handles. Finally, food should be served one course at a time, and there should not be too much food on the patient's plate nor too many objects on the table; items such as paper napkins can distract patients.

In the advanced stages of dementia, chewing food can take longer; often patients require help with swallowing in the form of cues such as verbal reminders, imitation of the process, or stroking the patient's throat or cheek. Neuromuscular problems in the pharyngeal musculature (eg, degenerative changes in corticobulbar tracks and cranial nerve nuclei) can lead to dysphagia and choking on liquids and solids.[155] Dysphagia usually develops gradually, progressing from occurrence with consumption of solids, then purées, and then liquids. If acute dysphagia develops, a thoughtful medical workup for reversible conditions should be performed.

Caloric intake in people with dementia often fails to meet metabolic requirements. As discussed previously, dysphagia may impede adequate oral intake. Other contributors to eating difficulties may include conditions associated with the mouth and gastrointestinal tract (eg, poor dentition, thrush, oral ulcers, delayed gastric emptying, fecal impaction, dry mouth); medication-related anorexia resulting from diuretics, beta blockers, digoxin, nonsteroidal anti-inflammatory agents, cholinesterase inhibitors, and amiodarone; and unrecognized symptoms such as depression, pain, and nausea.[156,157] Because of poor oral intake, slow-hand feeding, which takes considerable time (often more than 1 hour per meal), is often required.

When weight loss occurs or oral intake diminishes to an unacceptable level (often during an acute event such as pneumonia), the issue of feeding tube use often arises. Feeding tube placement for people with advanced dementia continues to increase despite the lack of literature supporting its use.[158-160] Reasons frequently cited for feeding tube placement include decreased mortality and aspiration, improved nutritional and functional status, and healing of pressure ulcers.[161] Although no RCTs exist that compare hand feeding with

tube feeding for end-stage patients with dementia, cohort and cross-sectional studies provide convincing evidence that tube feeding does not improve patient outcomes.[162] Mortality is high with or without feeding tube placement, with 30-day mortality averaging about 20%, 6-month mortality at 50%, and a median survival of 56 days.[158,163,164] Aspiration often continues after feeding tube placement, and many patients develop new aspiration after the tube is placed.[165] At the same time, feeding tube placement detracts from patient-focused care and is associated with frequent complications requiring transfer back to an acute-care hospital for additional interventions.[158] No studies published to date have assessed the impact on QOL of a feeding tube compared with slow-hand feeding. Many of the reasons cited for feeding tube placement are not supported by the evidence, and the burden of the intervention may outweigh the benefits of continued slow-hand feeding.

More efforts now focus on addressing goals of care related to feeding decisions before the question of a feeding tube arises. One approach has been to use a video decision support tool to facilitate advance care planning in cognitively intact people in the event that dementia develops and progresses to the advanced stage.[166] Compared with a verbal description, a video depiction was more likely to be associated with goals of care in advanced dementia that focus on comfort. Moreover, participants who watched the video had more stable preferences over time. Another approach currently being researched assesses the usefulness of a decisional support tool to facilitate advance care planning with surrogates regarding tube feeding in nursing home residents with advanced dementia.

Infection Treatment

Invariably a person with advanced dementia develops an infectious complication, usually a urinary-tract infection or pneumonia. One study found an in-hospital mortality of almost 20% in patients with advanced dementia receiving antibiotics, with a 6-month mortality rate of more than 50%.[32] During hospitalization, patients undergo many procedures that are reported to be painful, including daily blood draws, arterial blood-gas measurement, and IV-line placement. In addition, hospitalized patients with dementia remain at high risk for being placed in restraints to receive IV antibiotics and oxygen therapy.[32,167] Given these facts, it is not surprising that many dementia experts recommend that people with advanced dementia who have infectious complications not be hospitalized, which is the practice in other countries.[168] Moreover, compared with good palliative care (including antipyretics, analgesics, and oxygen), antibiotics do not improve patients' comfort, although they have been shown to improve survival for patients with advanced dementia and pneumonia.[169,170]

Hip Fractures

Hip fractures commonly occur in older adults with or without cognitive impairment. Bed-bound patients remain at risk for hip fracture, which can occur either during routine care (chair transfers, bathing, or changing soiled diapers) or spontaneously. The decision of whether to surgically repair a hip fracture in a bed-bound patient with severe cognitive impairment is challenging and requires consideration of the risks associated with hospitalization and surgical repair compared with palliative and hospice care. Surgery can be considered palliative because pain is likely to be less severe after the repair. The in-hospital mortality rate for fractured hip repair in patients with advanced dementia is relatively low (about 5%), but the 6-month mortality rate remains high (more than 50%).[32] People with dementia who have a hip fracture and who undergo surgical repair experience undertreated pain. In fact, 76% of patients with advanced dementia who were hospitalized for surgical repair did not receive a standing analgesic agent, according to two studies.[171,172]

The nonsurgical palliative approach to hip fractures for patients with end-stage dementia focuses on symptom management and prevention of complications. The predominant physical symptom after a hip fracture, particularly during routine care, is pain. As such, patients with hip fracture should not only receive adequate analgesia throughout the day to maintain comfort but also premedication before repositioning, transferring, and performing daily care activities such

CLINICAL SITUATION CONTINUED FROM P. 25

Margaret's Case Continues

Seven years after diagnosis, Margaret is wheelchair-bound. She is incontinent of stool and urine and utters 6 to 10 intelligible words a day. During the past month she has required more assistance with feeding and is pocketing food in her mouth. She was recently admitted for pneumonia, has developed a stage-2 sacral pressure ulcer, and has lost 15 pounds within the last 6 months.

Question Fourteen

A meeting is scheduled with Robert to discuss goals of care. He inquires about the possibility of gastrostomy tube placement because Margaret's sister had a feeding tube placed after having a cerebrovascular accident. Which of the following might be the best response?

A. "Don't you think she is tired of living?"

B. "A gastrostomy is a surgical procedure with some risks and discomfort."

C. "Tube feedings via a gastrostomy have not been shown to prevent recurrent aspiration or prolong life."

D. "Since there are other ways of keeping her comfortable, do you think she would want this now?"

Correct Response and Analysis

Responses B, C, and D could all be parts of a meaningful discussion of appropriate goals of care. Whether a gastrostomy tube is elected or not, plans should be put in place for palliating discomfort and avoiding burdensome hospitalizations for future infections. A hospice service should be explained and offered for continuing care. A is incorrect. Robert clearly cares for his mother, and implying that she is not worth more care is worse than unhelpful.

Question Fifteen

What are common complication(s) that occur as dementia progresses to end stage?

A. Acute infections

B. Pressure sores

C. Dysphagia

D. Hip fracture

E. All of the above

Correct Response and Analysis

E is the correct response. End-stage dementia from progressive neurodegeneration is associated with apraxia, dysphagia, and immobility that put people at high risk for medical complications. Common complications of end-stage dementia include pressure sores, infections (pneumonia and urinary tract), hip fractures, and malnutrition.

Question Sixteen

Feeding tubes in people with end-stage dementia have been shown to do which of the following?

A. Decrease hospitalization

B. Prevent aspiration pneumonia

C. Decrease mortality

D. Heal pressure ulcers

E. None of the above

Correct Response and Analysis

E is the correct response. Feeding tubes frequently are placed in people with end-stage dementia despite data suggesting little or no role for the reasons frequently cited. Feeding tubes have not been shown to decrease mortality and rates of aspiration pneumonia or improve functional status, pressure-ulcer healing, or nutritional status. Feeding tubes have not been shown to decrease the rate of hospitalization and, in fact, may increase risk because of complications associated with the placement and use of the tube.

Question Seventeen

Besides disease progression, which of the factors listed below may be associated with decreased oral intake in people with dementia?

A. Depression

B. Constipation

C. Dry mouth

D. Amiodarone

E. All of the above

Correct Response and Analysis

E is the correct response. Many conditions may contribute to declines in oral intake. Mouth-related issues include dryness, infection (thrush), ulcers, and poor dentition. Delayed gastric emptying, constipation, gastroesophageal reflux, and fecal impaction may also be associated with poor oral intake. Medications frequently associated with anorexia include digoxin, beta blockers, diuretics, and amioderone. Finally, unrecognized symptoms such as pain, shortness of breath, agitation, depression, and nausea may contribute to poor intake.

Continued on page 33

as dressing and bathing. Often, when opioids are required to adequately control a patient's pain, increased sedation may occur. Ultimately the risk-benefit ratio of opioid use must be considered in the context of the patient's QOL, goals of care, and limited life expectancy. One of the most common complications of hip fractures is the development of skin breakdown, which can occur despite the most rigorous preventive care, including frequent repositioning, getting patients out of bed, and optimizing nutrition. Given the poor prognosis of patients with hip fracture who have end-stage dementia, hospice referral should be considered and discussed with the patient's power of attorney independent of a decision about surgical repair.

Treatment of Comorbid Conditions

Several papers on inappropriate prescription of medication for older adult populations have been published. At the same time, disease-specific guidelines on appropriate pharmacotherapy continue to be created and revised. People with dementia have multiple morbidities that require numerous medications to comply with "current recommendations." Also, people with dementia take prescription and nonprescription drugs for their underlying neurodegenerative disease. As a result, these patients may be on a plethora of medications, many of which can interact and have additive side effects. For example, patients on cholinesterase inhibitors who develop urinary incontinence are likely to be placed on anticholinergics, which may lead to nausea and dry mouth, respectively, predisposing them to dehydration.

One approach to minimizing polypharmacy is to prioritize existing medications and consider discontinuing therapies that may no longer be providing clinical benefit consistent with the goals of care. To date, little attention has been given to if and when to discontinue otherwise appropriate therapy in people nearing EOL.[173] One frequently cited article suggests that a decision-making model should take into account remaining life expectancy, time until benefit is derived, goals of care, and treatment targets (ie, primary and secondary prevention and symptom control).[174] Using such an approach, healthcare providers can engage patients (when appropriate) and families in shared decision making about starting, stopping, or continuing therapy. Unfortunately, few studies are available to guide clinicians on which medications are least likely to provide clinically relevant benefits. This lack of information poses particular challenges when a medication may be offering some symptomatic benefit and the patient cannot relate their experience. For example, should NMDA receptor antagonists, which have been shown to improve patient and caregiver outcomes in moderate to severe AD, be discontinued in the more advanced stages of the disease? If discontinued, should the medication be tapered? What are the adverse effects of discontinuing the medication?

Hospice

Research suggests that patients dying of dementia receive suboptimal EOL care that includes poor symptom control and overly aggressive treatments. Despite research suggesting little or no benefit, many patients with end-stage dementia die with feeding tubes in place.[159,160] Compared with patients dying of cancer in nursing homes, dying patients with dementia are more likely to undergo bloodwork and be restrained.[149] Families may opt for extensive diagnostic workups, aggressive treatment of coexisting medical conditions, transfer to an acute-care facility with any change in condition, and cardiopulmonary resuscitation in the event of an arrest, which detracts from a palliative approach and has not been shown to prolong survival.[173]

Nursing home-, hospital-, and community-dwelling people with dementia are at risk for inadequate pain management. In one study, people with cognitive impairment who underwent hip surgery were given one-third the amount of opioid analgesic adminstered to cognitively intact patients.[171,172] Compared with cognitively intact nursing home residents in pain, cognitively impaired nursing home residents in pain were much less likely to receive analgesia.[84] Among community-dwelling people with dementia who could still report their pain experience, half of those who reported pain "on an average day" were not taking an analgesic.[176]

Many healthcare providers and families believe hospice care is the most appropriate care near EOL.[68] Moreover, no effective treatment of dementia exists, and patients exhibit considerable physical symptoms and self-care needs at EOL.[154] At the same time, caregivers experience a substantial burden and can benefit from additional support.[177] Despite the apparent need and the belief that hospice care is appropriate, a minority of patients—fewer than 10%—with advanced dementia die with the benefits of hospice services.[76]

Entry guidelines for enrollment into hospice for patients with advanced dementia are detailed in *UNIPAC 1*. The admission guidelines specify that an eligible patient with dementia must maintain substantial functional limitations (Functional Assessment Stage 7C: bed-bound, uttering few words, and requiring assistance with ambulation) and present with disease complications (eg, aspiration pneumonia, upper urinary-tract infection, septicemia, multiple decubitus ulcers [stage 3 or 4]), recurrent fever despite antibiotics, and inability to take in sufficient fluids and food to sustain life).[74] The functional assessment staging scale contains the following limitations[83]:
- It was not developed to predict life expectancy.

- It presents functional loss as an ordinal progression that is not necessarily the way in which the disease progresses.
- It is not derived from empirical data. In fact, one study found that hospice guidelines were better at predicting who would *not* die within 6 months than who would die.[83]

Although many studies support the benefits of hospice care for patients with cancer, few studies have been conducted among people with dementia. One study of nursing home residents, in which a majority were dying as a result of dementia, found those enrolled in hospice were twice as likely as nonhospice enrollees to receive regular treatment for pain.[178] Similarly, a nursing home study found that people dying with dementia on hospice were more likely to receive scheduled opioids for pain and directed therapies for dyspnea (oxygen, opioids, scopolamine, and hyoscamine); in addition, caregivers reported fewer unmet needs during the last 7 days of life compared with those who were not enrolled in hospice.[179] In another study of community-dwelling older adults with dementia who were dying, hospice enrollees were significantly more likely than nonenrollees to die in their location of choice—almost always at home—and less likely to die in a hospital. Caregivers of enrollees were also more likely to report care to be excellent or very good compared with caregivers of nonenrollees. However, the mean pain scores of hospice enrollees and nonenrollees were not significantly different, and on average caregivers for both groups reported the patient's pain at a moderate or higher intensity during the last 2 weeks of life.[178] On the whole, hospice improves the care of people dying with dementia, but more work is needed to better understand the assessment and treatment of physical symptoms that occur near EOL for patients across care settings, including the community, nursing homes, and hospitals.

Another scenario arises when caring for people with dementia: families often request hospice services for a loved one with advanced disease that is not yet severe enough to meet hospice eligibility criteria. A patient who is bedbound and incontinent with a recent pneumonia and can still utter more than six intelligible words per day is an example of such a patient. In such cases in which hospice admission is agreed upon, it is imperative for hospice and palliative care providers to document the reasons a patient's prognosis is considered to be shorter than 6 months (eg, recurrent aspiration pneumonia, accelerated weight loss, or recent stroke). Throughout the hospice course it is necessary that the team continue to document disease progression, and at recertification periods prognosis data must be reiterated, preferably with objective documented evidence of decline (eg, number of pneumonia episodes, number of centimeters of decreased triceps fold thickness, increased dependency with feeding).

Caregiver Issues

Compared with other chronic, disabling, life-limiting conditions, caring for a person with AD or related dementia poses unique stressors and challenges. With AD, the caregiver role usually lasts for many years and changes over time as the disease progresses. In addition to cognitive losses (eg, short-term memory, orientation, language difficulties, executive functioning), patients often develop personality changes and exhibit challenging behaviors such as agitation and aggression, loud vocalizations, and wandering. Over time, people with dementia require greater supervision during self-care activities and throughout the day and night to ensure adequate safety. Compared with other caregivers, those who care for people with dementia must provide greater assistance when transferring loved ones in and out of bed and with dressing, bathing,

toileting, and changing incontinence products.[19] Given these additional needs, caregivers of people with dementia report greater physical and emotional strain, take fewer vacations, have fewer hobbies, spend less time with other family members, and have more work-related difficulties such as having to reduce hours to part time, turn down promotions, and lose job benefits compared with caregivers of physically impaired older adults.[180]

Although caregiving provides many altruistic benefits for the caregiver, it comes at a considerable cost, particularly when caring for those with dementia. Caregivers of people with dementia have higher rates of depression and anxiety, and female caregivers report higher levels of depression and anxiety compared with male caregivers.[181-183] At the same time, caregivers are less likely to participate in preventive health behaviors and report experiencing mental and physical health problems arising from their caregiving.[180,181] Caregivers who reported mental and emotional strain had a 63% higher mortality risk than controls who did not report mental or emotional strain.[184] Given the increased strain on caregivers and the underlying vulnerability of people with dementia, it is not surprising that dementia is a risk factor for the mistreatment of older adults.

Caregivers face many difficult decisions as dementia progresses for their loved one. These decisions often come at a substantial cost for both themselves and the patient and may include taking over the patient's finances, taking away their car keys, and placing them in a nursing home. Certain patient and caregiver characteristics have been found to increase risk for nursing home placement for people with dementia.[185,186] Patient characteristics included being Caucasian, living alone, having greater functional and cognitive impairment, and exhibiting difficult behaviors. Caregiver characteristics included being older than 65 years and reporting a greater burden. Caregivers who reported that providing help to their relative made them feel useful, appreciated, and important were significantly less likely to place their relative in a long-term care facility. At the same time, caregivers who chose long-term care for their loved one did not report a decrease in depressive or anxiety symptoms; these effects were most pronounced among caregivers who were spouses, visited the patient more frequently, and reported less satisfaction with the help they received from others.

Many intervention studies have been designed to decrease caregiver burden and depression. These interventions focused on both the patient with dementia (eg, reducing care-recipient behaviors and dependency) and the patient's caregiver (eg, providing knowledge about caregiving and the relationship with the care recipient, available community resources and support, coping with and resolving feelings of depression and anxiety). Research suggests that using interventions that take into account caregiver strengths and abilities, target multiple domains, and focus on both members of the dyad (ie, the patient with dementia and the caregiver) have the largest impact and greatest success.[187,188] A randomized, controlled, and structured multicomponent intervention found the intervention arm was associated with lower rates of depression and greater improvement in QOL for Hispanic, Caucasian, and African American caregivers.[189] Caregiver health also improved; the intervention group reported better self-rated health, sleep, mood improvement, and physical improvement compared with the control group.[190] Despite these findings, the effect size of caregiver interventions may be smaller for those who care for people with dementia compared with other caregivers.[191] Local branches of the Alzheimer's Association can provide caregivers access to support groups and helpful educational courses. The Alzheimer's Association website, www.alz.org, offers a tremendous amount of educational material for caregivers.

The EOL and bereavement experience for caregivers of people with dementia living at home has recently been characterized.[177] Fifty percent of caregivers report spending 46 hours weekly helping their relative with ADLs and IADLs. More than 50% of caregivers reported feeling "on duty" 24 hours a day to perform their caregiving role. Before their relative's death, 43% of caregivers had substantial depressive symptoms, which declined significantly 3 months after the patient's death and within 1 year were significantly lower than when they acted as a caregiver. Complicated grief was more common among caregivers who had high levels of depressive symptoms and burden before their relative's death than in those who reported positive features of caregiving and who cared for relatives with greater cognitive impairment.[192]

Margaret's Case Concludes

After much discussion, Margaret is enrolled in a hospice program. She eats by slow-hand feeding with cues, is taking in minimal calories, and continues to lose weight. All of her medications including donepezil and memantine have been discontinued. She now is bedbound and completely dependent in all ADLs. She develops occasional periods of restlessness and fevers that respond to acetaminophen. She dies peacefully in the nursing home 4 months after hospice enrollment.

Question Eighteen

Which of the following statements support the enrollment of a person with dementia to hospice?

A. Being able to walk independently

B. Speaking two to three intelligible words a day

C. Aspiration pneumonia

D. Weight loss

Correct Response and Analysis

The correct responses are B, C, and D. The hospice criteria for dementia require the disease to be advanced enough to result in substantial functional limitations and severe enough to be associated with medical complications. From a functional standpoint, the patient must be unable to walk, dress, or bathe without assistance; have urinary and fecal incontinence; and be unable to speak six different intelligible words in a day. At least one medical complication should occur during the previous 6 months and include aspiration pneumonia, pyelonephritis, septicemia, multiple stage-3 or stage-4 pressure sores, fever despite antibiotics, or weight loss exceeding 10% of body weight.

Question Nineteen

What are the potential benefits of hospice enrollment for people with dementia?

A. More regular treatment for pain

B. Decreased hospitalizations

C. Prolongation of life

D. Increased support for family and professional caregivers

Correct Response and Analysis

The correct responses are A, B, and D. For people with a primary diagnosis of dementia, the hospice benefit compared with routine care provides superior patient and caregiver outcomes. Patients are more likely to die at home and are more likely to be prescribed medications for pain. Caregivers report higher satisfaction with care and receive additional support. Studies have not examined whether hospice enrollment for people with dementia is associated with a longer life expectancy.

Chronic Obstructive Pulmonary Disease

Epidemiology

COPD is unique among the major diseases in Western society; prevalence, burden of morbidity, and attributable mortality continue to rise.[193] In the general population in the Netherlands, for example, 3 of every 1,000 subjects are diagnosed with COPD per year.[194] The incidence increased rapidly with age and was higher in men than in women. One in 8 men and 1 in 12 women, being COPD-free at the age of 40, will develop COPD later in life.[194] In Dutch patients with very severe COPD, 26% died after 1 year of follow-up, whereas 2.8% died among the non-COPD subjects.[194]

The term COPD should be understood to include other commonly used terms such as chronic bronchitis and emphysema, all sequela of smoking-related inflammatory processes effecting large and small airways as well as lung parenchyma and vasculature. The destruction of lung tissue occurs because the primary

---

CLINICAL SITUATION

Edward and Betty

Edward is a 69-year-old retired machinist who has smoked for more than 50 years and lives with his wife, Betty. He has a known history of borderline hypertension and hypercholesterolemia but has been inconsistent about following up with his primary physician. He is not taking medication and continues to smoke despite repetitive urging to quit from his wife and two adult children. During the past 2 weeks Edward has been "fighting a cold" with worsening dyspnea on exertion, wheezing, and cough productive of scant white phlegm. He finally relented and went to the local emergency room, where a chest X ray revealed hyperinflated lungs and a flattened diaphragm without infiltrates. He was admitted with a COPD exacerbation and started on nebulizers and corticosteroids.

Question One

According to the body mass index, airflow obstruction, dyspnea, and exercise (BODE) Index, which of the following factors are predictive of a 2-year mortality of 30% to 40% in Edward?

A. Exercise capacity

B. Degree of airflow obstruction

C. Modified Medical Research Council dyspnea score

D. Body mass index (BMI)

E. All of the above

Correct Response and Analysis

The correct answer is E. Although clinical evidence is limited regarding the prognosis of COPD, several studies have examined predictors of increased mortality in people with COPD. The BODE Index was developed as a practical tool to measure a patient's degree of lung impairment, his or her perception of respiratory symptoms, and the ways in which the disease negatively affects the entire body as a system. BODE takes into account BMI, airway obstruction as measured by forced expiratory volume in 1 second (FEV_1), dyspnea (as measured by the MMRC dyspnea scale), and exercise tolerance (as measured by the 6-minute walk test). The BODE Index is thought to be a better predictor of COPD mortality than FEV_1 alone[221] (Table 9). As BODE scores increase, health-related QOL decreases.[222]

Continued on page 39

Table 9. Predictors of Increased Mortality for Patients with Advanced COPD

Increased Risk of Dying Within 12 Months (Proposed)[241]	6-Month Mortality of 30%-40%[206,225]	2-Year Mortality of 30%-40%[246]	Overall mortality predictors[247]

1. Best FEV$_1$ < 30% predicted
2. Increasing dependence on caregivers
3. Activity limited to a few steps without need to rest
4. Depression
5. No spouse
6. Recurrent hospitalization within the previous year
7. Associated chronic comorbid illness
	Using SUPPORT criteria: 2 of the following in hospitalized patients:
	
	1. Baseline PaCO$_2$ > 45 mm Hg
	2. Presence of cor pulmonale
	3. FEV$_1$ < 0.75 L
	4. Previous episode of respiratory failure within the last 12 months
		Highest quartile on BODE Index (ie, a score of 7-10)
		            Score
		B > 21 0
		   ≤ 21 1
		O FEV$_1$ 36%-49%.......2
		   FEV$_1$≤ 35%..............3
		D MMRC* score, 3.....2
		   MMRC* score, 4 3
		E Walks 150-249 m in 6 min....................2
		   Walks ≤ 149 m in 6 min....................3
			In multivariate analyses, the following factors were predictive of mortality:
			1. Increasing age
			2. Oxygen use
			3. Lower total lung capacity (% predicted)
			4. Higher residual volume (% predicted)
			5. Lower maximal cardiopulmonary exercise testing workload
			6. Greater proportion of emphysema in the lower-lung zone vs the upper-lung zone and lower upper-to-lower-lung perfusion ratio (P = .007)
			7. Modified BODE (P = .02)
			
			FEV$_1$ was not a significant independent predictor of mortality.

BODE: B, body mass index; O, degree of airflow obstruction; D, dyspnea; E exercise capacity; FEV$_1$, forced expiratory volume in 1 second; MMRC, Modified Medical Research Council; PaCO$_2$, partial pressure of carbon dioxide in arterial blood.

*MMRC score of 3 indicates a patient stops for breath at 100 yards or after a few minutes on level ground; MMRC score of 4 indicates a patient is too breathless to leave the house or is breathless while dressing or undressing.

inhaled toxins implicated in COPD (eg, first- or second-hand tobacco smoke, other inhaled environmental toxins) overwhelm natural local antiprotease defenses in the lungs. Patients with alpha-1 antiprotease deficiency who smoke are at particular risk for early-onset COPD.[195] Of the six leading causes of death in the United States, COPD is the only one to have increased steadily during the last 30 years.[196]

As one of the most common chronic diseases, COPD is a major cause of morbidity and mortality. In the United States some 150,000 patients with advanced COPD die each year; the overall death rate increased 8% between 2000 and 2005 (men increased 6% and women increased 11%).[197] In Canada COPD accounts for 4% of deaths annually and will result in more than 20,000 deaths per year by 2018.[198,199] Globally COPD is the fourth leading cause of death in the world, projected to become the third leading cause of death by 2020.[200,201] COPD affects more than 210 million people worldwide, and the average worker with COPD must retire at age 54.[202] Index admission mortality for an acute exacerbation of COPD usually is between 2.5% and 12%,[203-205] although the rates are somewhat higher if admission to an intensive care unit (ICU) is required.[206] Patients who survive hospitalization after an acute exacerbation of COPD often experience shortness of breath for the rest of their lives.[203] Compared with patients who have cancer, those with COPD spend increasing amounts of time in the hospital as their disease progresses.[207] In the last year of life, as many as 94% of patients with chronic lung disease experience dyspnea.[208] Compared with patients with lung cancer, patients with COPD are more likely to die with poor control of dyspnea.[209] For many, dyspnea is incapacitating.[208,210-213]

Neurophysiology of Dyspnea

Dyspnea is the sensation, usually unpleasant, of discomfort with breathing and manifests as one or more of the following: a sense of air hunger, increased work of breathing, and chest tightness. For participants in the Study to Understand Prognoses and Preferences for Outcomes and Risks of Treatment (SUPPORT) who died of COPD, dyspnea was the overriding complaint and was twice as common as the next most prevalent symptoms, pain and confusion.[203] Dyspnea is a significant source of disability for people with COPD (especially those with a low socioeconomic status[214]) and profoundly affects their QOL.[215] It is important to understand the mechanisms underpinning dyspnea as the basis for both conventional and novel approaches to symptom relief.

Dyspnea is not a single sensation; there are at least three distinct sensations including air hunger, work/effort, and chest tightness. Like pain, dyspnea has at least two distinct dimensions: sensory and affective. Sensory signals from the respiratory system are relayed to higher brain centers where they are processed and influenced by behavioral, cognitive, contextual, and environmental factors before shaping of the final sensation of breathlessness.[216] Recent neuroimaging studies suggest that neural structures subserving pain and dyspnea might be shared; consequently, the neurophysiological and psychophysical approaches used to understand pain might be applied to dyspnea research.[217] Sensory signals from the respiratory system are relayed to higher brain centers where they are processed and influenced by behavioral, cognitive, contextual, and environmental factors before the shaping of the final sensation of breathlessness. Each individual perceives, interprets, and reacts to the sensation of dyspnea from within his or her framework of history, experience, values, and beliefs—a dynamic that can result in a broad range of symptoms that affect physical, emotional, social, and spiritual domains. For the emotional domain, by using neural imaging,[216,218,219] healthcare professionals are beginning to understand the extent of limbic and paralimbic activity in patients with dyspnea that supports a treatment approach that considers the contribution of anxiety, fear, and other emotions along with mechanical issues based on hyperinflation.[220] When dyspnea is viewed as a mismatch between incoming afferent sensory information from the respiratory system and efferent motor activity or demands of breathing work, it is easier to understand why patients with advanced lung disease need more than a traditional, airflow-obstruction-focused, pharmacologic approach to symptom control.

Disease Trajectory of Severe COPD

The final years for patients with advanced COPD are characterized by progressive functional decline, poor QOL, and increasing dependence on informal caregivers and the healthcare system.[207] Ultimately many patients are faced with incapacitating breathlessness.[207,210-213]

The disease trajectory of COPD differs fundamentally from that of cancer.[223] Episodic exacerbations and incomplete recovery challenge the timing of any supportive intervention in accordance with patients' current needs. Studies conducted in the United States and Canada, including SUPPORT, have demonstrated that hospitalized patients with advanced COPD are more likely to receive technological interventions (often without the establishment of previous life-support preferences). Moreover, they often die in an ICU setting with greater symptom burden[203,209] and less input from other services such as palliative care.[207,223-225]

Patients with advanced COPD have special palliative care needs.[226] Patients recognize these needs.[227] There have been several calls for increased involvement from palliative care services for patients with advanced COPD,[203,209,224,228-231] including a position statement from the American College of Chest Physicians.[232] However, the benefit of this type of involvement, while intuitive, has yet to be carefully evaluated or fully implemented for patients with COPD.

Two key barriers exist between the time of a diagnosis of advanced COPD and the provision of quality EOL care: (a) the highly unpredictable disease trajectory discussed previously and (b) the fact that, in many cases, physicians have yet to help patients and their caregivers appreciate that COPD is a life-threatening disease.[203,225] Other impediments to provision of effective palliative care for patients with advanced COPD include patients' limited understanding of treatment options; barriers to effective communication resulting from attitudes of patients, physicians, and other caregivers[233-237]; and clinicians' limited ability to judge when palliative care services may be helpful.[238,239]

Compared with cancer, for which the terminal phase usually is recognized by both physicians and patients,[240] prognoses for patients with COPD are notoriously inaccurate; among the other 19 reasons for hospice referral in the United States, only dementia has a less-certain 6-month prognosis.[241] Common-sense guidelines have been proposed for identifying patients with advanced lung disease and minimal cardiopulmonary

reserve who can benefit from hospice and palliative care.[229] For example, the guidelines propose that patients would be eligible for hospice and palliative care if, despite an adequate trial of optimum available treatment, they have persistent troublesome symptoms or severe limitation of activity. These patients are likely to benefit from the specialized services offered by hospice programs because of their distressing symptoms or a severely limited performance status.[229] Another criterion would be COPD that has progressed to the point that a patient could die at any time of an ordinary intercurrent illness, such as bronchitis or pneumonia. These patients are likely to benefit from a careful assessment of their goals of care and advance care planning.

To help identify patients with COPD in the latter category who are at significant risk of dying within 1 year, Hansen-Flaschen[241] proposed a profile extrapolated from earlier studies of various predictors of mortality.[25,242-245] This approach has been adapted to develop an overview of prognostic predictors (Table 9).

Others have proposed use of the BODE Index.[246,247] However, even patients with the highest BODE Index quartile scores had a 2-year survival rate of 60% to 70%.[206,246] In addition to being associated with increased risk of death, health-related QOL decreases as BODE Index scores increase.[222] Mortality risk recently has been shown to increase with the frequency of each hospital admission for a COPD exacerbation.[248] These studies suggest that a combination of simple measures of disease severity can provide a reasonable indication of a likely poor outcome within 1 year.

Another study involving 609 patients with severe emphysema who were enrolled in the National Emphysema Treatment Trial confirmed that a combination of several factors, including the BODE Index, can help predict mortality among patients with severe airflow obstruction.[249] Despite these advances, it remains difficult to reliably predict which patients with COPD are likely to die within 6 months.[249]

Systematic Manifestations of COPD and Concomitant Comorbidities

Patients with severe COPD or recurrent exacerbations display increased markers of systemic inflammation including cytokines; acute-phase proteins; and circulating monocytes, neutrophils, and lymphocytes.[250] Although the origins of systemic inflammation remain unknown, there is growing evidence that inflammation is a driver of the disease process, which no longer can be viewed as being restricted to the lungs. This is supported by the fact that the increased mortality risk associated with the BODE Index incorporates nonpulmonary-related markers of

BMI and distance walked in 6 minutes. Examination of muscle tissue has found decreased aerobic enzyme activity, decreased type 1 fibers, decreased capillaries, the presence of inflammatory cells, and increased apoptosis.[251] A recent study of patients with COPD documented nonrespiratory impairment of function with poorer muscle strength, lower-extremity function, and exercise performance and mobility-related dyspnea after adjustments for lung function over a 2-year period, suggesting muscle fatigue rather than dyspnea is the primary factor limiting exercise tolerance.[252] In addition to impacting the disease course and clinical manifestation of COPD, the underlying inflammatory milieu may affect the presence and severity of frequently associated comorbid conditions such as cardiovascular disease (ischemia, arrhythmia, and heart failure), lung cancer, chronic kidney disease, osteoporosis, diabetes, and depression.[253]

CLINICAL SITUATION CONTINUED FROM P. 35

Edward and Betty's Case Continues

Edward is feeling much better and is discharged home with a bronchodilator. Because he was feeling well, he chose to cancel his follow-up appointment with his primary care physician. He resumes smoking and uses his bronchodilator on occasion when he becomes short of breath. During the next several months Edward notices gradual increasing dyspnea with exertion and a slight wheeze when climbing a flight of stairs. He finally gives in to his wife and schedules an appointment with his primary care physician, who prescribes an inhaled long-acting beta-agonist in combination with an inhaled corticosteroid. His oxygen saturation at rest is 95% on room air and falls to 92% with

exertion. A follow-up pulmonary function test reveals severe obstructive pulmonary disease. Edward's physician attempts to engage him in a conversation regarding the seriousness of his diagnosis and the implications for his future, but he responds, "I don't see the point in talking about this. I feel fine now." Betty adds, "He is stubborn and afraid to discuss these things. We are fortunate to have gotten him this far."

Question Two

Which of the following statements is true regarding use of combination therapy with a long-acting beta-agonist and inhaled corticosteroid for chronic management of Edward's COPD?

A. It will improve his survival.

B. It will decrease the incidence of pneumonia.

C. It will improve results on spirometry.

D. It will improve health-related QOL.

Correct Response and Analysis

The correct responses are C and D. A large RCT involving more than 6,000 patients compared the combination of salmeterol and fluticasone with placebo and with each agent alone.[259] Results failed to demonstrate a survival benefit with combination therapy, but health-related QOL and spirometry improved. In addition, the risk of pneumonia ($P < .001$) was increased with combination therapy or fluticasone alone versus placebo (see page 40).

Question Three

Which of the following is true regarding the use of oxygen therapy at this stage of Edward's illness?

A. He meets criteria by oxygen saturation.

B. He may experience less anxiety and depression.

C. Short-term oxygen use is recommended during exercise-induced desaturations.

D. If admitted to the hospital for an acute exacerbation, he should wear nasal prongs with a high flow rate instead of a Venturi mask.

Correct Response and Analysis

The correct response is B. Long-term oxygen therapy (LTOT) has a major effect on patients' lives. For some, the change in routine and restrictions associated with its use may be unacceptable. Others may experience less anxiety and depressive symptoms as they become more capable of enduring activity. With few exceptions, eligibility criteria for LTOT for most patients include an oxygen saturation at rest of ≤ 89% or a partial pressure of oxygen (PaO_2) < 55 mm Hg. There is little evidence to support use of oxygen therapy in persons with exercise-induced desaturations. Patients admitted to the hospital with an acute COPD exacerbation should be supplied oxygen through a Venturi mask to provide a controlled FiO_2. Use of nasal prongs can result in an inappropriately high FiO_2, which can lead to an increase in partial pressure of carbon dioxide ($PaCO_2$), hypoxic vasoconstriction, and reduced hypoxic drive.

Continued on page 44

Symptom Assessment and Control

The Dyspnea Ladder

Palliative care clinicians are familiar with the WHO pain ladder (see *UNIPAC 3*). Some authors propose incorporating a similar dyspnea ladder into the routine assessment of patients with progressing COPD (**Figure 1**).[254] As with any patient-physician relationship, clinicians should weigh the benefits and side effects of any medication on an individual basis.

Dyspnea Management

Despite optimal pharmacologic therapy targeting airflow obstruction, most people with severe COPD continue to have chronic, progressive dyspnea—a fact that reaffirms the need to identify evidence-based treatments for this burdensome symptom.

A number of interventions are available for dyspnea relief, including standard medical therapy with bronchodilators,[255] oxygen, surgical therapy (eg, lung-volume reduction surgery, lung transplant),[256] and use of opioids.[257] Despite use of such approaches, only 50% of patients with end-stage COPD obtain significant relief of dyspnea[212] and many live (and die) with incapacitating breathlessness.[213] At the same time, dyspnea is associated with substantial disability and diminished QOL (see *UNIPAC 4* for more on dyspnea relief).

Figure 1. The Dyspnea Ladder

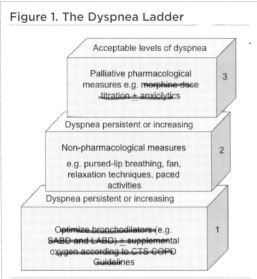

SABD, short-acting bronchodilator; CTS, Canadian Thoracic Society; LABD, long-acting bronchodilator.

From Rocker GM, Sinuff T, Horton R, Hernandez P. Advanced chronic obstructive pulmonary disease: innovative approaches to palliation. J Palliat Med. 2007;10:783-797.[254] © 2007 Mary Ann Liebert Publishers, Inc. Reprinted with permission.

Although a complete review of all available therapies is beyond the scope of this chapter, we will review some of the most important palliative care therapies for patients with severe COPD.

Conventional Pharmacologic Treatment for COPD

It is a given that all patients with advanced disease deserve optimal conventional therapy. Current Canadian Thoracic Society (CTS) guidelines for escalating the treatment for advancing COPD[258] are summarized in **Figure 2**.

In addition, evidence available[220,259] from large RCTs supports the use of a long-acting anticholinergic agent such as tiotropium[260] in addition to a combination of an inhaled long-acting beta-agonist and inhaled corticosteroid to decrease COPD exacerbations and improve health-related QOL for patients living with progressing COPD.[220,259,261] This benefit must be weighed against a meta-analysis that found long-term use of anticholinergics in COPD was associated with

Figure 2. Management of COPD

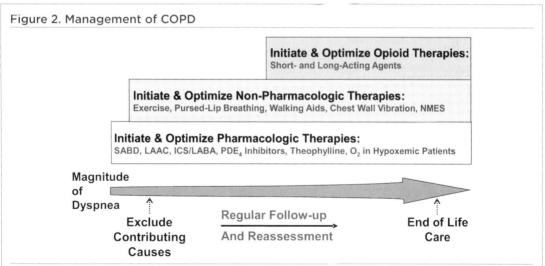

ICS, inhaled corticosteroids; LAAC, long-acting anticholinergics; LABA, long-acting beta-2 agonists; NMES, neuromuscular electrical stimulation; O_2, oxygen; PDE_4, phosphodiesterase 4; SABD, short-acting bronchodilators.

From Marciniuk D, Goodridge D, Hernandez P, et al. Managing dyspnea in patients with advanced chronic obstructive pulmonary disease: A Canadian Thoracic Society clinical practice guideline. Can Respir J. 2011;18(2):69-78.[258] © 2011 Canadian Respiratory Journal. Reprinted with permission.

a small but statistically significant increased risk of cardiovascular death—113 of 3,858 versus 62 of 3,369 (RR = 1.73 [1.27, 2.35]); $P < .01$) compared to placebo, respectively, although statistical significance was not reached for overall mortality.[2] Cessation of tiotropium did not seem to cause a rebound effect over 3 weeks of follow-up, suggesting these therapies can be safely discontinued if no longer consistent with goals of care.[263]

Bronchodilators

Inhaled bronchodilator therapy is a mainstay of dyspnea treatment for patients with COPD. Bronchodilators act by relaxing bronchial wall smooth muscle. They are available in various formulations and patient-activated devices (eg, metered-dose inhalers best used through spacers such as aerochambers), dry-powder inhalers (eg, diskhaler, turbuhaler), and wet nebulizers (mostly for patients who cannot use other devices). Guidelines from the American College of Physicians (ACP), American College of Chest Physicians (ACCP), American Thoracic Society (ATS), and European Respiratory Society (ERS) for 2011 suggest the following:

- clinicians prescribe monotherapy using either long-acting inhaled anticholinergics or long-acting inhaled beta-agonists for symptomatic patients with COPD and FEV_1 < 60% predicted. (Grade: strong recommendation, moderate-quality evidence.) Clinicians should base the choice of specific monotherapy on patient preference, cost, and adverse effect profile.
- clinicians may administer combination inhaled therapies (long-acting inhaled anticholinergics, long-acting inhaled beta-agonists, or inhaled corticosteroids) for symptomatic patients with stable COPD and FEV_1 < 60% predicted. (Grade: weak recommendation, moderate-quality evidence.)[264]

Systemic therapies that target bronchodilation are less successful. Theophylline is not recommended because it has relatively weak bronchodilatory effects and uncertain effects on diaphragmatic function,[265] and it can have significant systemic side effects.

Corticosteroids

Precious few data suggest that systemic corticosteroids are beneficial in the long term for chronic, stable COPD, although randomized trials continue.[266] The Global Initiative for Chronic Obstructive Lung Disease statements on COPD recommend that systemic steroids not be used for this condition because of their significant side effects and the lack of compelling data suggesting significant benefit.[267] Inhaled corticosteroids certainly have far fewer adverse effects, but data indicating they benefit patients with chronic, stable, severe COPD also are limited. A randomized trial by Burge and colleagues (the ISOLDE trial) suggested that patients with moderate or severe COPD who receive inhaled corticosteroids experience a very small but statistically significant benefit in health-related QOL, with a slightly slower decline over several years than patients randomized to placebo.[268] As a result, inhaled corticosteroids are a reasonable adjunct treatment for patients with severe COPD who have frequent exacerbations.

Combination of Bronchodilatation and Inhaled Corticosteroids

For many patients with advanced COPD, the combination of a long-acting beta-agonist and an inhaled corticosteroid can prove more beneficial for symptom management and QOL than either agent alone.[269] Calverley and colleagues reported that the combination of salmeterol and fluticasone failed to provide a survival benefit in a large RCT involving more than 6,000 patients that compared this combination with placebo or with either agent alone. Other facets of living with COPD improved, however, including health-related QOL and spirometry, although pneumonia risk was higher ($P < .001$) with combination therapy or fluticasone alone versus placebo.[259]

Long-Term Oxygen Therapy

Inhaled bronchodilators and anti-inflammatory medications are, in themselves, not sufficient to provide symptom relief as COPD progresses; other therapies must come into play. As patients in the later stages of COPD adapt to the limitations of the disease, oxygen often is prescribed to those who are eligible. Eligibility criteria may vary in different settings, but in general a non-smoking patient with an oxygen saturation at rest of ≤ 89% or a PaO_2 < 55 mm Hg is a suitable candidate. Similarly, patients with proven pulmonary hypertension secondary to COPD or with cor pulmonale should use LTOT for 15 to 24 hours each day. There is little evidence to suggest any long-term benefit from short-term oxygen use secondary to exercise-induced desaturations.[270] As a single therapy, LTOT can have a major effect on patients' lives by changing their routines and cause restrictions that necessitate new rhythms in life; LTOT also can be viewed as an advantage—a way to survive, endure, and adapt—and ultimately may be tolerated by some users.[199] Some patients have described a negative image of living with LTOT because of its interference with their desire to appear healthy. Others have described the dominance of technical thinking and sustained work the treatment required from them. Such negative effects can be ameliorated with greater compassion and understanding from healthcare providers.[271]

LTOT as an adjunctive therapy might improve patients' QOL by lessening their anxiety and depression and enhancing emotional function and mastery, but for some it is unacceptably limiting and intolerable.[272]

Use of Oxygen During Acute COPD Exacerbations

The use of oxygen during acute exacerbations of COPD, especially for patients with baseline hypercarbia, needs to be carefully controlled. In this situation, oxygen at high flow rates through nasal prongs can be dangerous. It often is forgotten that the hospital oxygen supply arrives at a concentration of 100% at the bedside, and, to achieve a known concentration of oxygen inhaled by the patient, a Venturi mask must be used to supply a controlled FiO_2 of 24% or 28%. If nasal prongs are used, the FiO_2 that reaches the nares approaches 100% at high flow rates, and at any flow rate the ultimate FiO_2 depends on dilution of supplied oxygen by the amount of air breathed in at the same time. An inappropriately high FiO_2 can cause an increase in $PaCO_2$ through several mechanisms, including reduced hypoxic drive, which causes a lower-minute ventilation and less clearance of CO_2. This can be particularly dangerous when the work of breathing is increased as a result of bronchoconstriction and sputum retention. A second and perhaps more common effect is the disturbance of pulmonary hypoxic vasoconstriction. When pulmonary hypoxic vasoconstriction is reversed under the effects of high inspired and alveolar FiO_2, blood is diverted to underventilated areas of the lung, which causes additional ventilation/perfusion mismatch that further exacerbates the elevation of $PaCO_2$. Displacement of CO_2 from more oxygenated hemoglobin into plasma also occurs (the reverse of the Haldane effect). For all of these reasons, it is best to avoid or limit the use of nasal-prong oxygen during acute exacerbations of COPD, especially for patients with hypercarbia. For these patients it is better to instead rely on delivering oxygen via Venturi mask to achieve a saturation of peripheral oxygen (SpO_2) of around 89% to avoid the deleterious effects discussed above while also providing a safe level of oxygenation.

Supplemental Oxygen for Mildly Hypoxemic Patients

Supplemental oxygen administered via nasal cannula can greatly improve exercise tolerance and dyspnea, even for patients with mild hypoxemia (those patients who do not meet the traditional criteria for LTOT of an SpO$_2$ > 89%). The administration of both compressed air[273] and supplemental oxygen to a patient with mild hypoxemia with COPD (ie, oxygen saturaton > 89%) has been shown to relieve dyspnea.[274] A therapeutic trial of oxygen for dyspnea relief may be indicated for treatment of persistent dyspnea. The CTS states

Continuous oxygen therapy for hypoxemic COPD patients reduces mortality, and may reduce dyspnea in some patients. The CTS has previously recommended that patients with advanced COPD who are hypoxemic at rest receive long-term continuous oxygen therapy because of a mortality benefit. Oxygen therapy may also provide symptomatic benefit by reducing dyspnea when administered at rest to hypoxemic patients with advanced COPD (grade of recommendation 2B). There is no evidence to support the routine use of supplemental oxygen to reduce dyspnea in nonhypoxemic patients with advanced COPD. There appears to be little benefit from supplemental oxygen on QOL in patients with advanced COPD.[258]

The authors of a 2011 Cochrane Review, "Symptomatic Oxygen for Non-Hypoxaemic Chronic Obstructive Pulmonary Disease," concluded that

Oxygen can relieve dyspnoea in mildly and non-hypoxaemic people with COPD who would not otherwise qualify for home oxygen therapy. Given the significant heterogeneity among the included studies, clinicians should continue to evaluate patients on an individual basis until supporting data from ongoing, large randomised controlled trials are available.[274]

CLINICAL SITUATION CONTINUED FROM P. 40

Edward and Betty's Case Continues

Edward's health begins to deteriorate over the next 4 years. He is finding it increasingly difficult to maintain his ADLs as the result of persistent dyspnea with exertion despite maximum medication management. Betty has taken over lawn-mowing and other household chores he is no longer able to perform. Edward managed to quit smoking and has decided to forgo his monthly poker games with his friends who continue to smoke. He is no longer able to participate in hobbies he loves such as fishing and bowling due to respiratory symptoms. Recently he was discharged from the hospital after his second admission this year for COPD exacerbation with superimposed pneumonia. He is now using home oxygen which has helped, but he is also experiencing anxiety when he suddenly becomes short of breath after climbing eight stairs to his master bedroom. Betty is concerned that Edward is becoming depressed and more isolated due to limitations in his functional status and social life. Edward's pulmonologist contacts a palliative care consultant to evaluate his needs. The palliative care team performs a comprehensive assessment to identify the best approach to Edward's dyspnea (see *UNIPAC 4*).

Question Four

Which of the following is true regarding the addition of opioids to treat Edward's dyspnea?

A. Nebulized opioids are more effective.

B. Recommended starting doses of oral opioids for dyspnea are higher than those used for pain treatment.

C. Low-dose opioids, when used correctly, are not associated with respiratory depression.

D. Studies have shown the most common adverse effect of opioid therapy in people with COPD is delirium.

Correct Response and Analysis

The correct response is C. Several studies have confirmed that opioids, when started at low doses and titrated appropriately, improve the symptoms of dyspnea with minimal side effects. Starting doses for stable opioid-naïve patients generally are recommended to be lower than doses commonly used for pain management. Long-acting opioids have similarly demonstrated benefit, with constipation being the most common reported adverse effect. To date, studies have not demonstrated improved efficacy in the use of nebulized opioids over oral preparations for dyspnea.

Question Five

In addition to oral opioids, which of the following nonpharmacologic strategies show the best evidence for the management of Edward's dyspnea?

A. Neuromuscular electrical stimlulation in the lower extremity

B. Rolling walker

C. Pursed lip breathing

D. Acupuncture

Correct Response and Analysis

The correct responses are A, B, and C. The CTS and a recent Cochrane review found several nonpharmacologic interventions to be effective in managing dyspnea in patients with COPD.

Neuromuscular electrical stimulation on the calves and quadriceps in bedbound patients improves dyspnea, muscle strength, and performance of daily tasks. Rolling walkers are thought to decrease dyspnea when users assume a leaning posture with arm support on the device. Pursed-lip breathing decreases dyspnea through improved gas exchange by decreasing respiratory rate and increasing vital capacity. There is insufficient evidence to support the use of acupuncture in managing dyspnea from COPD.

Question Six

Which of the following statements is false regarding the value of pulmonary rehabilitation for Edward's condition?

A. Self-management programs are associated with a decrease in the number of COPD exacerbations.

B. Self-management programs are associated with a reduction in hospital admissions.

C. Self-management programs are associated with an improvement of dyspnea

D. Patients undergoing pulmonary rehabilitation demonstrate an improvement in anxiety.

Correct Response and Analysis

The correct answer is A. Patient self-management education as part of pulmonary rehabilitation emphasizes giving patients the knowledge and skills necessary to make behavioral changes to improve health outcomes. A recent review found these programs were associated with reduced hospital admissions and improvement of dyspnea, but there was insufficient evidence to show benefit in reduction of COPD exacerbations, emergency department visits, and change in exercise capacity. Outpatient pulmonary rehabilitation programs have yielded multiple benefits including improvement in exercise capacity, dyspnea, QOL, anxiety, depression, and sense of control over the disease.

Continued on page 50

Other Pharmacologic Approaches
Opioids

Opioids are an important addition to the treatment of dyspnea for patients with severe COPD who have been maximally treated with bronchodilators and other therapies; the role of opioids has been recognized in professional society position statements on COPD.[275] A number of randomized trials and a 2011 meta-analysis[257,258] suggest that oral opioids reduce the sensation of dyspnea, but their use is associated with some side effects. For example, a randomized trial involving administration of sustained-release morphine for 4 days showed reduced dyspnea scores but increased constipation despite laxative treatment.[276] A recent open-label study of primarily COPD patients who were opioid naïve and experienced significant dyspnea examined the feasibility of initiating long-acting morphine at 10 mg daily with subsequent increases of 10 mg weekly up to 30 mg daily.[277] The response rate, defined as at least a 10% improvement in dyspnea on a visual analog scale, was 63%, with a number needed to treat of 1.6 and a number needed to harm of 4.6. The most common adverse effect was constipation, and none of the 83 participants were hospitalized for respiratory depression, delirium, or decreased level of consciousness. A meta-analysis also suggests that although oral and parenteral opioids are effective,[257] nebulized opioids are ineffective,[257] a conclusion supported by a report in 2004.[278] It is important to remember that the opioid studies considered in the systematic review[257] were all short term. Although long-term studies on the effects of opioids in advanced COPD are scarce, these drugs nevertheless should be considered, not only for EOL situations but also for stable patients with COPD whenever their breathlessness is severe and continues despite maximal bronchodilator therapy. Low-dose opioids do not appear to cause significant respiratory depression.[276] Several studies assessed within the systematic review[257] attest to the absence of adverse effects on blood gases.[279] The Australian and Canadian guidelines on COPD both include guarded recommendations for considering opioids for severe dyspnea.[280] Physicians should commence opioid therapy conservatively for such stable patients (see *UNIPAC 4*). This starting dose can gradually be titrated to the point of satisfactory relief of dyspnea. Lower starting doses might be needed for elderly patients and those with a very low BMI. Longer dosing intervals may be appropriate for patients with renal insufficiency. Higher starting doses and more rapid escalation can be appropriate for severely distressed patients whose goals emphasize comfort more than life-prolongation. As always, clinicians should anticipate and be prepared to deal with the most common side effects including constipation, nausea, and transient sedation.

Patients who experience an acute, unremitting dyspnea crisis need a comprehensive, expert, multidisciplinary evaluation. Their treatment should be aggressive and may include escalating doses of oral or parenteral opioids (see *UNIPAC 4*). Benzodiazepines are less effective and more sedating but may be considered a third-line agent when opioids and nonpharmacologic measures have not been successful.[281]

Nonpharmacologic Approaches
Other Modalities

In 2011 the CTS released an evidence-based clinical practice guideline for the management of dyspnea in patients with advanced COPD who continue to experience symptoms despite standard therapies; this guideline mirrors the findings of a Cochrane review.[258,282] It includes pharmacologic therapies of short- and long-acting bronchodilators (beta-agonists and anticholinergics), inhaled corticosteroids, and theophylline preparations as well as nonpharmacologic therapies of pulmonary rehabilitation (see below) and oxygen therapy (as discussed above). Nonpharmacologic interventions considered as part of the review (and elsewhere)[283] were the use of a fan, neuromuscular electrical stimulation, assist devices, pursed-lip breathing, meditation, relaxation, and behavioral techniques. The use of neuromuscular electrical stimulation in calves and quadriceps in patients with severe COPD (including mostly bedbound patients) has been associated with improved dyspnea, muscle strength, and performance of daily tasks. Rolling walkers decrease dyspnea, possibly through forcing users to assume a forward-leaning posture along with arm support on the device. Pursed lip or diaphragmatic breathing also decreases dyspnea, possibly through improved gas exchange by decreasing respiratory rate and increasing vital capacity.[284] Chest wall vibration also appears to be effective.[282] Insufficient evidence is available to support the use of handheld fans to decrease breathlessness; a 2010 RCT with an active control group could not prove the effectiveness of these fans.[285] Both the practice guidelines and the Cochrane review contend that insufficient evidence exists to support the use of acupuncture, acupressure, distractive auditory stimuli, relaxation, and psychotherapy, although other sources recommend these interventions in certain circumstances.[283]

Lung reduction surgery[249] and lung transplants are becoming more common but will not be useful to most palliative care patients. Newer bronchoscopic lung volume reduction techniques may show promise as alternative treatments for select patients with COPD undergoing consideration for lung transplantation.[286]

Pulmonary Rehabilitation
The American Thoracic Society and the European Respiratory Society define pulmonary rehabilitation as

...an evidence-based, multidisciplinary, and comprehensive intervention for patients with chronic respiratory diseases who are symptomatic.... Integrated into the individualized treatment of the patient, pulmonary rehabilitation is designed to reduce symptoms, optimize functional status, increase participation, and reduce healthcare costs through stabilizing or reversing systemic manifestations of the disease.[287]

Four large professional societies reaffirmed their recommendation that pulmonary rehabilitation should be considered for any patient with symptomatic COPD who does not achieve optimal physical and social performance despite optimal pharmacologic treatment.[264] Participants in pulmonary rehabilitation typically attend 6 to 12 weeks of individualized exercise training, self-management education, nutritional counseling, and psychosocial support sessions. There is substantial evidence for improvement in dyspnea, exercise tolerance, functional capacity, health-related QOL, and healthcare utilization with pulmonary rehabilitation, particularly in COPD.[288] Additional benefits include decreasing anxiety and depression and an improved sense of control over the disease.[251] Lacasse and colleagues performed a systematic Cochrane review that included a large number of well-conducted RCTs of pulmonary rehabilitation in COPD. They found both statistically and clinically meaningful improvements in functional exercise capacity (assessed using the 6-minute-walk distance) and chronic dyspnea (assessed using the dyspnea domain of the Chronic Respiratory Questionnaire).[289] Despite the substantial physiological and clinical benefits of pulmonary rehabilitation in COPD, it remains underused as a therapy for a number of reasons, including insufficient availability of facilities and inability of patients to travel to participate in these programs because of distance or cost considerations. Home-based pulmonary rehabilitation can be effective and, like patient self-help groups, helps maintain exercise tolerance and QOL over time.[290,291] Pulmonary rehabilitation may be less effective for patients with severe COPD who are chairbound or bedbound because of their COPD.[215]

Homecare and Self-Management Education

Patient self-management education is a core component of pulmonary rehabilitation and goes beyond simply providing information to patients in didactic lectures. The emphasis is on teaching patients the knowledge and skills necessary to make behavioral changes that lead to improved health outcomes.[292]

The pulmonary rehabilitation setting provides opportunities to address patients' educational needs. It has been known for some years that patients with COPD want information about their disease and management options.[224,225,293] A 2007 Cochrane systematic review examined the efficacy of self-management education for patients with COPD.[294] Heterogeneity existed among the 14 trials, which included limiting the ability to conduct some of the meta-analysis. The review found that self-management programs were associated with a significant reduction in at least one hospital admission compared with routine care (odds ratio, 0.64 [0.47, 0.89]). Not surprisingly, the effect size was largest for people at highest risk for rehospitalization. QOL also was significantly improved in the self-management arm compared with routine care, but the clinical significance was uncertain. Dyspnea as measured on the BoRG scale (0-10, with higher scores indicating greater breathlessness) significantly improved on average by -0.53 (-0.96, -0.10). No beneficial effects were found between self-management and routine care in the number of exacerbations, ED visits, and exercise capacity.

Living Well with COPD is a prototypical self-management education program that was tested in a Canadian multicenter RCT involving 191 patients.[288] The program contains seven modules. Several of the modules address symptom management, but the program does not address EOL care. The program includes the following modules:

- Module 1 presents educational material providing basic information about COPD, breathing and coughing techniques, energy conservation, and relaxation exercises.
- Module 2 educates patients on preventing and controlling symptoms with inhalation techniques.
- Module 3 includes techniques to recognize an acute exacerbation and initiate a plan of action to manage it.
- Module 4 presents information on adopting a healthy lifestyle.
- Module 5 is about leisure and travel.
- Module 6 is a home exercise program.
- Module 7 presents information about understanding indications and implications of home LTOT.

The program was presented to patients in their homes by trained educators during a 7- to 8-week period. The program presentation was combined with a customized action plan for managing acute exacerbations of symptoms and providing ongoing case management support by telephone. Most of the patients were elderly and had advanced COPD with $FEV_1 < 1$ L; almost 50% experienced severe dyspnea. Patients in the intervention group had significantly fewer ED and unscheduled physician visits, fewer hospital admissions, and improved health-related QOL compared with patients receiving conventional care.[288] As with any multifaceted intervention, it was not clear which facets of the intervention (education, counseling, provision of support services, action plan for dealing with acute exacerbations) were most effective and responsible for improved outcomes.

However, few of the patients involved were near EOL—the 1-year mortality rate in the control and intervention groups was 9% and 5%, respectively.

Self-management programs that focus on the needs of patients with severe COPD with high symptom burden and likelihood of death are sorely needed, and such programs will hopefully be the focus of future research.[295]

Multifaceted Interventions for Dyspnea
Moving beyond individual therapies, Bredin described an intervention for dyspnea for patients with lung cancer.[296] In the United Kingdom, Booth and colleagues described a *breathlessness intervention service* (BIS) and its influence on patients living with intractable dyspnea.[297] The BIS model is based on four consultations. During the first consultation, a patient meets with a physician and physiotherapist. Severity of dyspnea and QOL are assessed and recorded. Patients are asked to indicate three goals they would like to achieve through the BIS. Needs of their informal caregivers are assessed at the same time. The second consultation occurs about 1 week later, and a tailor-made exercise program is planned. Patients receive advice about breathing exercises, use of pursed-lip breathing, use of fans to direct cool air,[298] body positioning, and help with daily activities. Referrals to other specialists are made at this visit. The third assessment is performed by the physiotherapist, who telephones the patient's home at about the third or fourth week to check on progress and answer questions. The final assessment occurs 4 to 6 weeks after the initial assessment to allow for feedback, symptom measurement, and ongoing support plans.

A phase 1 qualitative study by Booth and colleagues that assessed the BIS intervention showed that patients and families valued being listened to, receiving empathy, and having someone they could call when they were frightened; patients and families also noted the importance of "looking at what was possible rather than dwelling on what had been lost."[297] Even the recognition by the BIS team that caregivers of patients with dyspnea were doing all they could proved to be valuable, according to the feedback received from family members. It is important that this promising intervention be evaluated in future studies and in other settings.

Noninvasive Ventilation in End-of-Life and Palliative Care

The addition of noninvasive ventilation (NIV), mechanical ventilation via mask, to medical management has become the standard of care in the treatment of patients with moderate to severe exacerbations of COPD who have resultant acute hypercapnic respiratory failure. In this situation, NIV reduces the risk of intubation, length of hospital stay, and risk of mortality.[299] The role of NIV in chronic, stable COPD, specifically as a treatment offering potential palliation, is much less certain. At EOL, the rationale for providing assisted ventilatory support (eg, NIV) should be grounded firmly in the ability to provide comfort and relief of dyspnea. Two early (1992 and 1994) small case series reported that NIV can reduce dyspnea and preserve autonomy in appropriately selected patients who decline invasive ventilatory support.[300,301]

There has been a recent resurgence in interest in assessing the effectiveness of NIV for patients who have compromised mechanical ventilation. Such patients include those with advanced COPD living at home or in hospice settings who develop acute respiratory failure requiring hospital admission or patients on palliative care units of acute-care hospitals. The use and effectiveness of NIV for patients with acute respiratory failure and do not attempt resuscitation (DNAR) status remains controversial. Some of the controversy may be attributable to a lack of clarity about goals of care. NIV can be used for some patients to reverse an acute deterioration, with the aim of prolonging the patient's survival throughout hospitalization and returning to his or her previous level of functioning. In other cases NIV can be used for palliation of patients at EOL to relieve dyspnea or allow patients time to get their affairs in order.[302] Within the context of setting agreed-upon goals of care, there should be an understanding among the patient, caregivers, and the healthcare team that NIV can be withdrawn to allow a natural death if it cannot achieve the hoped-for aims within an accepted time frame. If the patient, caregivers, and healthcare team believe the benefits outweigh the burden and if the healthcare team has sufficient experience with NIV, then NIV may have a beneficial time-limited role.[303] It is essential to determine the goals of care when considering NIV use (or any other intervention) for patients with advanced COPD.[304]

CLINICAL SITUATION CONTINUED FROM P. 45

Edward and Betty's Case Continues

With the help of the palliative care team, Betty and Edward are able to express their concerns about their finances, psychosocial support, spiritual issues, and care planning. Edward is started on morphine elixir, 2 mg every 6 hours and as needed along with a bowel regimen, in addition to his inhalers and oxygen, for dyspnea management. The dose is gradually titrated up to 5 mg every 4 to 6 hours. His exercise tolerance and mood improve significantly with participation in a 12-week outpatient pulmonary rehabilitation program. He successfully traveled on two fishing trips with his son Brian and started playing poker again with his friends. Edward has slowly opened up about his fears. He says he was raised in the Catholic faith and "feels guilty" that he stopped going to church 10 years ago but declines meeting with a chaplain. He also is worried about Betty and how she will fare financially and emotionally if he dies. He has told his family that he does not want to be resuscitated if his condition deteriorates and if his physicians believe he cannot be successfully weaned from a ventilator.

One year later Edward is lost to follow-up, his symptoms progress, and he presents to his primary care physician with increasing pedal edema. His condition is diagnosed as cor pulmonale, and he is started on oral diuretics but is unhappy with the associated urinary frequency. He easily becomes short of breath with minimal exertion and spends much of his day on the couch watching television and refusing to accept visitors. He is eating poorly and has lost 10 pounds. Betty is feeling stressed and gets upset when Edward does not eat or consistently take his medications. One evening Edward develops sudden dyspnea that is unresponsive to oral morphine. He presents to the ED in respiratory distress and is started on NIV. After a tenuous overnight stay in the ICU, Edward's symptoms improve and he is transferred to the general medical unit. When the palliative medicine team arrives the next morning, Edward becomes emotional, stating, "Why is this happening to me? I am so tired of being a burden on everyone!" Betty and their son disclose they have been frustrated because he has not been willing to discuss his illness with his family. They ask if anything can be done at this point to improve Edward's condition and prevent him from having to be rehospitalized.

Question Seven

According to the literature, which of the following are potential barriers to adequate advance care planning among patients like Edward?

A. Inadequate information on the disease course when he received his diagnosis

B. Difficulty in defining what "end of life" means for a COPD patient

C. Lack of clarity in who should be driving the advance care planning discussions

D. All of the above

Correct Response and Analysis

The correct response is D. Healthcare providers identify several barriers when trying to initiate advance care planning for patients with COPD, including inadequate information about the course of COPD at the time of diagnosis, lack of consensus on who should initiate these discussions and in which care setting, concern that advance care planning would hinder patients from participating in self-management, and difficulty in defining what EOL means to people with COPD.

Question Eight

Which of the following statements is true regarding hospice eligibility for Edward at this point in his illness?

A. He currently does not meet criteria because he has never been intubated.

B. He meets criteria due to unintentional weight loss.

C. He does not meet criteria for COPD because he has cor pulmonale.

D. He meets criteria due to decreased functional capacity.

Correct Response and Analysis

The correct responses are B and D. Current published hospice eligibility guidelines (see *UNIPAC 1*) do a poor job of predicting 6-month mortality in people with COPD. Nevertheless, patients with any of the following factors should be considered potential candidates for hospice if they are aligned with the patient's goals of care (eg, comfort measures at home rather than recurrent hospital care): (a) disabling dyspnea at rest, poor or unresponsive to bronchodilators, resulting in decreased functional capacity, fatigue, and cough; (b) progression of end-stage disease as evidenced by increasing ED or ambulatory physician visits or hospitalizations for infections or respiratory failure; (c) hypoxemia at rest on room air and on supplemental oxygen; (d) cor pulmonale and right heart failure secondary to pulmonary disease; (e) unintentional and progressive weight loss of more than 10% in the last 6 months; (f) resting tachycardia (pulse over 100 beats per minute).

Continued on page 56

Palliative Care Needs

Studies using qualitative methods to focus on the needs of patients with advanced COPD have been conducted in the United States, Canada, and Europe.[305] In the United Kingdom, for example, analysis of postbereavement interviews with family members after 209 deaths resulting from COPD clearly indicated there was insufficient surveillance and inadequate provision of both primary and specialist care during the year before death.[212] In the United States, Curtis and colleagues described the need for physicians skilled in communication who can discuss a broad range of topics about EOL care, including informing patients about their prognosis and what dying might be like.[306] Heyland and colleagues reported the key elements of quality EOL care identified by 434 seriously ill hospitalized patients in Canada (including 118 patients with COPD).[307] The patients with advanced COPD at high risk for 6-month mortality (and their caregivers, when available) completed questionnaires to identify the aspects of EOL care most important to them and to report their level of satisfaction with those aspects of care.[225,308] For the patients with advanced COPD, the most important unmet needs concerned symptom relief, not wanting to be a burden to family, receiving adequate information (including benefits and risks of treatments), having a physician available to discuss COPD and answer questions in a way they can understand, and having adequate health services after being discharged from the hospital.[225] Similar themes (poor symptom control, need for information, and the impact of symptoms on patients' and caregivers' lives) have emerged from studies of advanced COPD in the United Kingdom.[211,309]

Recognizing the Influence of Anxiety and Depression

Anxiety and depression are common in patients with COPD—each effects as many as 40% to 50% of patients—and are much more prevalent than in the general population.[231,310-312] Unfortunately, these symptoms often go untreated and are associated with a poorer QOL.[313,314] It is important to achieve a better understanding of the high prevalence of COPD-related mood disorders that have been reported during the last 20 years[315-317] and the roles of gender and disease severity in the onset of anxiety and depression.[318,319] In addition to reducing the severity of depression, depression treatment can have beneficial effects on many aspects of living with COPD, including alleviation of dyspnea and other physical symptoms.[320] No compelling evidence supports the use of anxiolytics specifically for dyspnea.[281] However, cognitive or behavioral therapy decreases anxiety and depression in COPD and may be helpful for treating dyspnea in the context of severe anxiety.[321-325] In a large multicenter study conducted in Scandinavia, the prevalence of anxiety for patients with COPD was nearly 50%.[319] Anxiety has been associated with poorer health in patients with COPD, including poorer exercise performance, greater functional limitations, and a higher risk of COPD exacerbation.[326] Other studies have indicated that depression is an independent predictor of mortality in advanced COPD.[327,328] In addition, one study found depression to be associated with a patients' preference to have potentially life-sustaining treatments withheld; another study did not, suggesting that such preferences may need to be reassessed after treatment of or improvement in depressive symptoms.[329,330]

Data collected from family members in London during postbereavement interviews after the occurrence of 209 deaths attributable to COPD clearly indicated the burden of anxiety and depression among the patients before their death; low mood was reported for 77% of patients, and anxiety or panic attacks affected 53% of the patients, according to family members' reports.[212] In a series of stories about emotional vulnerability, Bailey described a "dyspnea-anxiety-dyspnea cycle" after an acute exacerbation of COPD as a common theme in interviews with 10 patients and their families.[210] She related how simple, everyday frustrations can induce anxiety, which is followed by increased breathlessness and more anxiety and more breathlessness, with no easy way of breaking this cycle without seeking help or rushing to the local ED. Nevertheless, treatments traditionally limited to the hospital setting also can be provided in patients' homes by nurse practitioners or by paramedics linked to emergency services. Other studies have described the potential value of the pulmonary rehabilitation setting as a venue in which to help patients learn strategies to reduce anxiety and depression.[331] Care providers' recognition of the psychosocial needs of patients with COPD[332] will need to be acknowledged more often as a key facet of the provision of quality care in the advanced stages of COPD.

See *UNIPAC 2* for additional information on assessing and managing anxiety and depression in COPD.

Improving Communication and Reducing Delays in End-of-Life Decision Making

Advance care planning is particularly important in COPD because the disease course typically is characterized by overall gradual decline punctuated by acute exacerbations that increase the risk of dying. In the United States, most patients enrolled in pulmonary rehabilitation programs welcome discussions about advance care planning and mechanical ventilation,[333] yet such discussions occur for fewer than 20% of patients with advanced COPD.[334] It has been known for years that patients with COPD request information regarding diagnosis, the disease process, treatment options, prognosis, what dying might be like, and advance care planning.[293] As of 2011, however, this rarely occurs in the United States.[335] Physicians should be prepared and adequately trained to ascertain their patients' wishes. Patients often believe their physicians do not understand their EOL care preferences[198,333] and want them to initiate EOL care discussions,[336] yet many physicians remain reluctant to do so.[230]

Healthcare providers who care for patients with COPD identify several barriers when trying to initiate advance care planning; these barriers include inadequate information given to patients about the course of COPD at the time of diagnosis, a lack of consensus on who should initiate these discussions and in which care setting, concern that advance care planning would hinder patients from participating in self-management, and difficulty in defining what EOL means to patients with COPD.[337] A recent review article proposed an approach to advance care planning for patients with COPD, and the approach mirrors standard techniques taught in palliative care.[338] The first step involves preparing for the conversation at an appropriate time and place when all people who are relevant to the patient are present. The second step is the discussion itself, which should review the diagnosis and the transition points over the course of the illness. These points include the initial presentation, escalation of treatments, disease exacerbations and hospitalizations, functional decline, initiation of LTOT, lack of additional treatment options beyond symptomatic management, and the dying process itself. As part of this conversation the patient's values and goals are discussed and EOL preferences elicited. The role and value of a surrogate decision maker are also discussed. The conversation reinforces the goals of preventing suffering and nonabandonment. Patient and family concerns and questions are addressed. After the discussion, the conversation is documented and reassessed with subsequent changes in health status.

It is an unfortunate reality that informal caregivers often do not have or have not been provided with adequate information, and they fail to recognize that patients might die from COPD[212]—another factor that is likely to limit their willingness to discuss the essential but difficult topic of addressing future needs while there is opportunity to do so. Beyond providing a much needed timely and empathetic discussion in a suitable setting as described above, clinicians should also consider recommending decision aids to help patients who face EOL choices.[237,339,340] For example, use of a structured decision aid concerning mechanical ventilation helped 33 patients with severe COPD make a choice; 74% of the patients chose to forgo mechanical ventilation.[339] Given the deficiencies in the decision-making process and in quality of care for advanced COPD, appeals for increased access to palliative care services are justified.[208,209,224,229-231]

Hospice

In 2009 lung diseases accounted for 8.2% of hospice admissions and were the fourth most common noncancer diagnosis.[341] As with other noncancer diagnoses, hospice criteria for COPD do a poor job of predicting who will die in 6 months.[342] Criteria for severe chronic lung disease and hospice eligibility generally include

- disabling dyspnea at rest, poor or unresponsive to bronchodilators, resulting in decreased functional capacity, fatigue, and cough
- progression of end-stage disease as evidenced by increasing ED visits or hospitalizations for infections or respiratory failure or increased physician visits prior to admission.

Supportive features are

- hypoxemia at rest on room air and on supplemental oxygen
- cor pulmonale and right heart failure secondary to pulmonary disease
- unintentional and progressive weight loss of more than 10% in the last 6 months
- resting tachycardia (pulse over 100 beats per minute).

Although hospice in general has been found to be effective for improving EOL care, studies are needed to directly compare outcomes for people with COPD who are enrolled and not enrolled in hospice.

Spiritual Issues

Numerous studies in the United States suggest that most patients want to discuss spiritual or religious issues with their physicians.[343,344] Studies from Europe suggest that religion may be an important determinant of the care patients receive.[345] Patients with COPD report that most physicians do not discuss their spiritual concerns with them, and they rate the quality of physician communication about spirituality as poor.[306] Several reviews offer approaches physicians may take when discussing religion with patients,[346,347] and validated measurement tools are now available.[348,349]

One important goal of spiritual care in EOL contexts is for the patient and family to be able to achieve a sense of peace, which can be facilitated by providing a hospitable interpersonal space for exploring illness-related concerns, fears, and hopes. Feelings of guilt due to self-inflicted disease can be a major source of suffering in patients with COPD.[350] The main components of a spiritual care approach include providing a compassionate presence, listening actively, giving unconditional acceptance, validating emotions, and providing supportive counseling if needed. Attention to the spiritual dimensions of suffering in COPD is a way to facilitate patients' trust in the healthcare team, closure, strengthening of relationships, and counteracting fears of abandonment and burden-related anxiety—all of which are issues that patients with COPD report as being important to them.[351-355] Puchalski and colleagues suggest that healthcare providers have an ethical obligation to provide opportunities for patients and their families to explore illness-related spiritual distress.[356] Lo and colleagues recommend opening such discussions always mindful of personal comfort levels and expertise constraints.[347] Referral to trained, credentialed chaplains on staff in major tertiary care centers is an available and relevant option for patients for whom religious, theological, and psychospiritual themes are prominent in their experiences with disease.[347,353,357] Chaplains are comfortable with the topic and can engage in extensive discussions with patients regarding prognostic uncertainty, emotional vulnerability, preparations for dying, and personally meaningful redirection of goals of care.[358] Despite the fact that palliative care, by definition, includes attention to all sources of suffering, including psychospiritual, patients and families continue to be underserved in this important area of EOL care.[351,353,356]

Caregiver Issues

Although caregiver burden is often highlighted in the cancer community,[359-362] measurement of burden is becoming an important part of palliative care studies.[363,364] Interventions are being tested for effectiveness.[365-367] Qualitative studies have underscored the extent to which both informal caregivers and patients with COPD suffer.[210,231,368,369] The demands on caregivers that are connected with the physical, emotional, social, spiritual, and financial aspects of caring for patients with chronic illness are compounded by a real or perceived lack of support. Patients in the late stages of COPD often are housebound yet receive little or no support from community health services.[213,224] Fear of being a burden on family is a major concern of patients living with advanced COPD,[225] which serves as an additional rationale for providing support services to informal caregivers.

Overall, the theme of loss is central to the care of patients with COPD. Multiple losses are reported by informal caregivers in COPD, including social isolation, boredom, tension in the relationship with the patient, fatigue, resentment, restriction of personal freedom, anger, helplessness, guilt, depression, difficulty sleeping, anticipatory grief, and loss of identity.[369-372] Because the fear of being a burden to family has been identified as a major concern of patients living with advanced COPD, it prompts these questions: Do those providing informal care for patients with advanced COPD actually feel burdened by this task and, if so, what causes their distress, and are there interventions that could ameliorate their suffering? Would caregivers of patients with advanced COPD benefit from the provision of an approach to care that concurrently considers both their needs and those of the patients? Although there is an obvious need for such interventions and approaches, research into palliative or other innovative models for caring for informal caregivers of patients with COPD is in its infancy.

Currently care of advanced COPD is primarily and reactively focused on physical symptoms and acute exacerbations. Families often are left to grapple with significant unrecognized and unaddressed psychosocial and spiritual suffering, including the ever-present threat of impending death.[373] This is particularly true when the death of the patient surrounds an ICU stay. In one prospective study, posttraumatic stress disorder (PTSD) was present in 14% of caregivers, while 18.4% reported depressive symptoms.[374] Family characteristics associated with either PTSD or depression were female gender, knowing the patient for a shorter amount of time, and discordance between family preferences for decision making and actual decision-making roles. Families with psychological symptoms reported that access to a counselor and spiritual services might have provided some benefit. A better understanding of informal caregiving experiences and burdens in other settings is sorely needed to guide appropriate development of COPD-specific services aimed at better support for informal caregivers.

The complexity of caregiver burden makes the burden difficult to measure in any exact or predictive way. Qualitative studies aimed at increasing the depth of understanding of complex health-related phenomena such as caregiver burden have been proposed.[375-377] Qualitative studies can produce a richness and depth that uniquely augment the use of standardized quantitative scales, such as the Caregiver Reaction Assessment.[369,375,376]

Ultimately, healthcare providers need to know whether and how much caregivers benefit from selected palliative interventions provided to patients with COPD. Although some benefit has been seen in populations that include patients with diagnoses other than COPD,[378] it is important to assess the feasibility and efficacy of a team-managed approach for the support of caregivers of patients with COPD in diverse settings.[379]

Conclusion

The provision of quality palliative care to patients with COPD and their families needs to begin early in the disease process and should not wait until dyspnea becomes intractable in the terminal stages. Patients, families, primary-care clinicians, pulmonary specialists, and the palliative care team can work in synergy to provide both traditional optimal medical therapy and more innovative approaches to palliative care.[379,380] A particular emphasis should be placed on informed decision making that recognizes patients' resuscitation preferences and other EOL issues. Patients and their families can benefit from improved self-management and a planned approach to addressing dyspnea (including use of the dyspnea ladder) and COPD exacerbations, use of hospice and palliative care services, and novel concepts such as a BIS or crisis intervention at home.

CLINICAL SITUATION CONTINUED FROM P. 51

Edward and Betty's Case Concludes

With the assistance of the palliative care team, Edward and his family elect to enroll in a home-based hospice program. His goal is to try to live long enough for the birth of his first grandchild. He is started on long-acting opioid therapy and an antidepressant. He also received training in cognitive behavior therapy to assist with the anxiety related to his dyspnea. Both Edward and Betty have been receiving counseling from the hospice social worker and chaplain and have found their marriage to be stronger than ever. Six months later, Edward dies peacefully with his family, including his newborn grandson, at his bedside.

Congestive Heart Failure

Definition and Diagnostic Criteria

Heart failure is a major cause of death for which mortality rates are increasing. Because symptom burden, disease therapy, and illness trajectory in heart failure can be quite different from those in other patient populations, it is important to understand palliative care for this population.

Heart failure is a clinical syndrome that results from a structural or a functional cardiac disorder that hinders the ability of the ventricle to fill with or eject blood. The most common clinical manifestations of heart failure are dyspnea, fatigue, exercise intolerance, and volume overload. Because heart failure is a clinical syndrome, diagnosis is based on a combination of the historical findings of dyspnea and fatigue with physical evidence of low cardiac output or volume overload. Although many patients with heart failure present with peripheral edema and symptoms of pulmonary congestion (eg, rales on examination), some patients with chronic volume overload may not have pulmonary congestion on examination because of a proliferation of pulmonary lymphatics. Moreover, some patients with primarily low cardiac output present with signs of shock (eg, cool extremities, impaired cognition). For these reasons, care should be taken when evaluating a patient for heart failure, and a heart failure diagnosis should not be ruled out on the basis of the absence of peripheral edema or rales on examination. Structural abnormalities alone (low ejection fraction [EF] or valvular heart disease in the absence of current or prior heart-failure symptoms) are insufficient when diagnosing heart failure. In addition, serum B-type natriuretic peptide levels can be elevated in conditions other than heart failure and are sensitive to other biological factors.[382] For that reason, these levels should never carry more diagnostic weight than clinical signs and symptoms of heart failure, and they have little or no role in the hospice and palliative care setting. There is no single test for the diagnosis of heart failure. It is a clinical diagnosis based on a careful history and physical examination.

The clinical syndrome of heart failure may result from disorders of the pericardium, endocardium, myocardium, or great vessels. The underlying cause of this cardiac dysfunction can be quite variable. In most patients, heart failure results as sequelae of coronary artery disease including myocardial infarction (MI), valvular heart disease, or long-standing hypertension. However, many other disease processes can contribute to the development of heart failure. Most patients with heart failure have symptoms resulting from impaired left ventricular (LV) function. Disorders of LV function causing the clinical syndrome of heart failure can range from a normal-sized LV with a normal EF to a dilated LV with a low EF.

Patients with a normal EF previously were classified as having diastolic heart failure or diastolic dysfunction. Patients with a low EF are classified as having systolic heart failure. Most therapy for heart failure is based on clinical trials of patients with systolic heart failure, although the numbers of clinical trials of patients with heart failure who have a normal EF is increasing. It is estimated that as many as 20% to 60% of patients with heart failure have a normal EF. These patients may have varied natural histories and may require treatment strategies different from those for patients with a low EF. It is thought that impaired ventricular compliance is a major cause of these

CLINICAL SITUATION

Paul

Paul is a 43-year-old morbidly obese gourmet chef who received his first heart failure diagnosis in his mid-thirties after he developed symptoms of fluid congestion following an acute myocardial infarction (MI). He initially sought medical care for his heart failure. With therapy consisting of an angiotensin-converting enzyme (ACE) inhibitor, a beta blocker, low-dose diuretics, and modest sodium and fluid restriction, he was free of symptoms for several years. Paul's biggest difficulty in coping with his illness was compliance with his diuretic regimen. He found it difficult to take the diuretics while working in the kitchen because of his frequent need to use the bathroom. In addition, his lifestyle and love of gourmet food made it difficult for him to comply with fluid restriction and a low-sodium diet. He also had trouble controlling his weight. After changing jobs and moving to a different location, he lost his health insurance and stopped following up with his cardiologist. He eventually stopped taking all of his heart medications. He has been living this way for several years, with dyspnea occurring occasionally during his normal daily activities.

Question One

According to the New York Heart Association (NYHA) Classification for Congestive Heart Failure, what functional class is Paul currently in?

A. Class I

B. Class II

C. Class III

D. Class IV

Correct Response and Analysis

The correct answer is B. All patients with heart failure traditionally are classified using the NYHA classification system based on their symptoms in relation to daily activity. Patients may move through all functional classes based on response to treatment with heart failure therapies. While on medications, Paul was symptom-free, which put him in Class I. After discontinuation of therapy he experienced symptoms with ordinary activity and subsequently progressed into Class II.

Question Two

Which of the following statements is true regarding Paul's risk for burdens of heart failure as his disease progresses?

A. He is less likely to develop physical symptoms, depression, and poor spiritual well-being compared to patients with advanced cancer.

B. His rate of functional decline in the advanced stage will be slower compared to people dying of cancer.

C. He is at significant risk for impairments in memory and executive dysfunction.

D. Anxiety is most likely to be his most common symptom.

Correct Response and Analysis

The correct answer is C. A cross-sectional study found that patients with stable heart failure had impairments in verbal memory, psychomotor speed, and executive function compared to those without heart failure.[381] A is incorrect because patients with heart failure experience a similar symptom burden compared with persons with advanced cancer. B is incorrect because patients who are dying with heart failure experience a more rapid decline in functional ability compared with patients dying with cancer. D is incorrect because pain and dyspnea are the most common reported symptoms in patients with heart failure.

Continued on page 62

patients' clinical syndrome. Most of these patients have a long history of hypertension. This type of heart failure is most common in elderly patients, particularly elderly women.[382,383]

Classification of Patients with Heart Failure

Traditionally, all patients with heart failure have been classified using the NYHA Classification for Congestive Heart Failure system according to their heart failure symptoms (**Table 10**). Because symptoms can improve with heart-failure therapy, patients are able to move between these designated classes of heart failure. For example, a patient with a new heart failure diagnosis after an acute MI might be dyspneic with minimal activity (NYHA Class III) but could enjoy sufficient improvement in those symptoms after several months of heart failure therapy if he or she no longer experiences dyspnea with ordinary activity (NYHA Class I). Moreover, many patients with heart failure remain on their medical therapy even if they have shifted to a lower NYHA classification.

For these reasons, the ACC/AHA staging system was developed in 2001 to complement the NYHA Classification system.[382] The ACC/AHA staging system (**Table 11**) emphasizes the development and progression of heart failure and does not allow patients to move to an earlier stage. Only patients in stages C through D actually have heart failure and fit into the NYHA classification. The ACC/AHA staging system is useful for determining appropriate therapies for patients. Patients in stages B and C are managed with medical therapies and occasionally cardiac resynchronization therapy (CRT) or implantable cardiac defibrillators (ICDs). More invasive therapies such as heart transplant, chronic IV inotropes, or a left ventricular assist device (LVAD) are considered for stage D patients. These patients are most often referred for palliative care.

Table 10. NYHA Classification System for Heart Failure

NYHA FUNCTIONAL CLASS

Chart	Description
I	Symptoms' only with more than ordinary activity
II	Symptoms with ordinary activity
III	Symptoms with minimal activity
IV	Symptoms at rest

NYHA, New York Heart Association.

*NYHA symptoms include fatigue, palpitations, or dyspnea.

Table 11. ACC/AHA Staging System for Heart Failure

Stage	Description
A	At high risk for developing HF but no structural heart disease or symptoms of HF
B	Structural heart disease but no signs or symptoms of HF (includes asymptomatic patients with low EF, valvular disease, LVH, or prior MI)
C	Structural heart disease with prior or current symptoms of HF
D	Refractory HF requiring specialized interventions such as heart transplant, chronic inotropes, or LVAD

ACC/AHA, American College of Cardiology/American Heart Association; EF, ejection fraction; HF, heart failure; LVAD, left ventricular assist device; LVH, left ventricular hypertrophy; MI, myocardial infarction.

In contrast to the ACC/AHA staging system, the NYHA classification is useful for capturing how the patient is functioning at a given point in time. Most current prognostic information about heart failure is based on the NYHA classification system. Clinicians caring for patients with heart failure should be familiar with both classification systems. Both systems apply to patients with both systolic heart failure and heart failure with normal EF.

Epidemiology

As mentioned previously, heart failure is a common disease that causes significant morbidity and mortality. It can adversely affect patients'

QOL with respect to both physical and emotional symptoms and can pose a significant financial burden to the patient and to society as a whole.

Incidence and Prevalence

At age 40 the estimated risk of developing heart failure sometime during one's lifetime is 1 in 5, and the risk is doubled for those with poorly controlled hypertension.[384] In 2004 an estimated 57,700 patients in the United States died of heart failure, and during the period between 1994 and 2004 the death rate from heart failure had increased by 28%.[384] This increase in the rate of heart failure deaths has been attributed in part to improved survival after an acute MI. A patient can now survive an acute MI and then go on to develop heart failure. Also, heart failure primarily is a disease of elderly patients. As the population ages, increasing numbers of patients are developing heart failure. The incidence of heart failure approaches 10 in 1,000 after age 65, and approximately 80% of hospitalized patients with heart failure are 65 years or older.[384] Heart failure is the single most frequent cause of hospitalization in people 65 years or older, and approximately 4.9 million Americans have this diagnosis.[385] Moreover, it is estimated that as many as 5% to 10% of patients with heart failure have end-stage disease.[386]

Burdens of Heart Failure

Symptoms

Clinically stable patients with heart failure appear to experience a similar symptom burden as patients with advanced cancer.[387] That is, people with NYHA class II, III, and IV heart failure reported a similar number of physical symptoms, amount of depression, and spiritual well-being as patients with lung and pancreatic cancers. Reports of each of these domains did not vary between patients with heart failure with an EF over 30% compared with 30% and lower.

However, among patients who reported lower heart-failure-specific health status, overall symptom burden, depression, and spiritual well-being was significantly worse compared to patients with heart failure who reported better health status or had advanced cancer. Patients with heart failure report significant life disruption, social isolation, symptoms, and uncertainty about prognosis and symptoms. A 2010 cross-sectional study[381] also found that medically stable patients with heart failure had significant impairments in verbal memory (total and delayed recall), psychomotor speed, and executive function compared with a control group. Of note, the differences reported were considerable and likely associated with clinical relevance although not necessarily indicative of a progressive neurodegenerative disease. Unfortunately, neuroimaging was not available to evaluate whether cerebrovascular burden could explain the observed differences in cognition between the two groups.

The etiology of heart failure symptomatology is not completely understood. However, recent work suggests the underlying physiologic changes that accompany heart failure substantially contribute to a patient's symptom experience; these changes are depicted in **Figure 3**.[388] Activity of the renin-angiotensin-aldosterone system, increased catecholamines, and proinflammatory cytokines contribute to heart failure–associated anorexia and cachexia along with cardiac, respiratory, and skeletal musculature atrophy. These later changes contribute to fatigue, dyspnea, mood changes, and diminished exercise capacity. Also, sleep-disordered breathing is extremely common in heart failure, which can further worsen neurohormonal and inflammatory changes.

Patients who are dying of heart failure have significant physical symptoms.[382,390] One large US study of caregiver perceptions of patients

Figure 3. Schematic Etiology of Heart Failure Symptoms

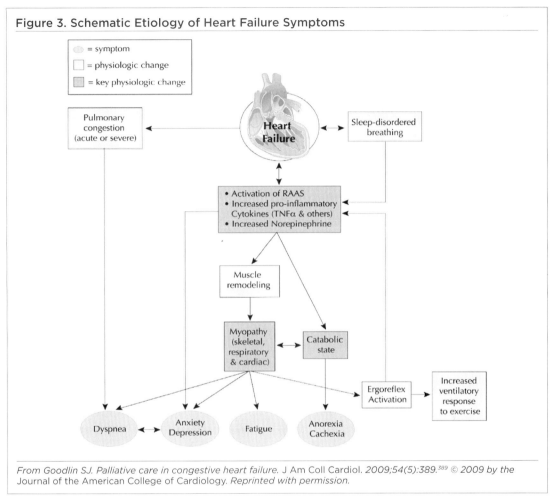

From Goodlin SJ. Palliative care in congestive heart failure. J Am Coll Cardiol. *2009;54(5):389.*[389] © 2009 by the Journal of the American College of Cardiology. *Reprinted with permission.*

dying of heart failure found that, during the last 3 days of life, 63% of caregivers perceived the patient was experiencing severe dyspnea, and 41% perceived the patient to be in severe pain.[204] In another study, friends and families of patients dying of heart disease were asked about symptoms the patient experienced during his or her last year of life. Seventy-eight percent of respondents reported the patient had pain, 61% reported the patient had dyspnea, 59% reported the patient had low mood, and 30% reported that the patient had anxiety. Patients also were reported to have experienced significant mental confusion, insomnia, anorexia, constipation, and nausea and vomiting. The patients for whom symptoms were reported to have been severely distressing or who were more reliant on the care of others were more likely to be perceived as having a poor QOL.[391] Furthermore, it is known that patients dying of heart failure experience a functional decline sooner than patients dying of cancer.[25] For patients with heart failure, overall QOL is poor[392] and involves multiple comorbidities,[393] especially for elderly patients.[394] Suffering is more intense than for patients with cancer,[391] and it is prolonged.

Financial Burden

The direct and indirect costs of heart failure in the United States in 2010 were estimated at $39.2 billion,[395] and costs are rising.[384] Increasing costs are the result of the increasing prevalence of heart failure and the high cost of heart-failure therapies. A mainstay of therapy for heart failure is hospital admission for treatment of volume overload. In fact, heart failure is a leading cause of hospitalization and hospital readmission within 30 days of discharge in people older than 65 years. The estimated average cost of admission for heart failure is $5,912, and the number of admissions has dramatically increased—from 399,000 in 1979 to 1,106,000 in 2006.[384,395] Invasive therapies for heart failure such as ICDs and CRT devices also are costly. It was estimated that in 2005 Medicare spent $30,000 for each ICD implanted.[396] The average cost of insertion of the CRT device has been estimated at $34,000.[397]

For patients with stage D heart failure, the ACC/AHA recommends evaluation for heart transplant or insertion of an LVAD. The total cost of a hospital stay for heart transplant and LVAD insertion has been reported at $145,000 and $198,000, respectively.[398] The cost of implanting newer devices seems to be lower.[399] Although the number of patients who receive heart transplants will remain relatively stable because of limited organ availability, the number of patients who receive LVADs may increase because this therapy, which first was developed as a bridge to heart transplantation, now has FDA approval for patients ineligible for a subsequent transplant as "destination therapy" (in which a patient can receive an LVAD as the final phase of therapy rather than as a bridge to cardiac transplantation).

Heart failure is a chronic, costly debilitating illness. Patients with heart failure live longer and have a better QOL on medical therapy, but the therapy can be expensive. Moreover, gradual functional decline can lead to significant disability that causes many patients to require extra nursing care at home or placement in a long-term care facility.

Heart failure is an illness of exacerbations. Many patients experience frequent exacerbations that require hospitalization. Frequent hospitalizations can be disruptive and can contribute to the financial burden of illness in both the direct costs of hospitalization and lost wages for patients and caregivers. The impact of advanced heart failure on caregivers can be profound. Data from the SUPPORT study of patients with acute heart failure exacerbations indicated that the likelihood of a family member having to quit work was 13%, and about 25% of families lost most of their savings.[400]

CLINICAL SITUATION CONTINUED FROM P. 58

Paul's Case Continues

Eventually Paul began to experience more prominent symptoms of congestion, including peripheral edema, fatigue, and dyspnea with minimal exertion (NYHA Class III heart failure). His symptoms became so debilitating that he presented to an ED and was admitted to the hospital in florid heart failure. At that time he was found to have an EF of 30% and modest renal insufficiency. He responded well to IV diuretics and was placed on an ACE inhibitor, beta blocker, and oral diuretic regimen with fluid restriction of 2 L per day. An ICD was placed as a prophylaxis against any possible lethal ventricular arrhythmias. Over the next few years Paul was readmitted several times with volume overload despite adherence to outpatient medical therapies, including the addition of spironolactone and vasodilators (NHYA Class IV). More recent admissions required temporary treatment with IV inotropes. Paul queried whether he would be a candidate for an LVAD or cardiac transplantation.

Question Three
Which of the following statements is true regarding ICD placement in Paul?

A. Indications include an EF lower than 35% with an estimated survival of at least 1 year.

B. Having an ICD placed at the NYHA Class III stage likely will reduce heart failure hospitalizations.

C. Paul is not at risk for an ICD pocket infection if the device is implanted.

D. Paul is likely to report an improvement in functional status after placement of the ICD.

Correct Response and Analysis
The correct answer is A. ICDs are implantable devices that sense potentially fatal arrhythmias and automatically defibrillate to restore normal sinus rhythm. The ACC/AHA recommends these devices should not be considered for patients expected to live less than 1 year who have poor functional capacity. Although ICD placement may prolong survival by avoiding sudden cardiac death, no studies have found reduced heart failure mortality,[401] improvement in QOL or function, or reduction in hospitalizations for heart failure symptoms. Several complications may occur including infections and pocket erosions after implantation and pain and psychological trauma from inappropriate firing. Careful consideration must be given to the role of these therapies in patients who are nearing EOL because burden eventually may outweigh expected benefits.

Question Four
Which of the following statements are true regarding LVAD therapy?

A. LVADs are not approved by the FDA for destination therapy.

B. The survival after continuous flow LVAD placement is about 5 years.

C. LVAD therapy improves exercise capacity.

D. People with LVAD implants report a poor QOL.

Correct Response and Analysis
The correct answers are A and D. Due to the scarcity of available organs, an increasing number of patients are undergoing LVAD placement as a final phase of therapy rather than a bridge to cardiac transplantation. Studies have shown that patients receiving LVADs have an improvement in functional capacity, QOL, and survival. Patients eligible for LVAD therapy have a life expectancy that ranges between 6 months and 2 years, depending on chosen interventions.[402] As technology of these devices continues to advance, the role of invasive therapies in palliative management of advanced heart failure is likely to increase.

Continued on page 70

Disease Trajectory and Management
Disease Course
The disease course of advanced heart failure is difficult to describe because of continued advancements in heart-failure management. Even for highly symptomatic, functionally limited patients, aggressive medical and device-based heart-failure therapy can have dramatic benefits. The widespread use of such therapies influenced the natural history of the disease. For a few patients who reach the end stages of the disease, interventions such as cardiac transplantation and

LVAD are options that potentially can improve survival and QOL.

Data from large patient registries and therapeutic trials show that heart failure is a chronic illness marked by exacerbations and periods of recovery. Unlike patients with cancer who usually maintain good functioning until relatively late in their disease course, patients with heart failure experience significant disability related to their symptoms throughout much of the course of their illness. These periods of stable disability are interrupted by periods of acute decompensation that often are amenable to therapy. Patients often can return to their previous level of functioning after an exacerbation. Eventually, however, they begin to lose ability to function during exacerbations. Many patients die of heart failure during an acute exacerbation,[403] but it is difficult to predict which of these exacerbations is likely to be fatal (**Figure 4**). Some patients also die suddenly of ventricular arrhythmias. However, improved medical therapies and the implantation of ICDs have significantly reduced the incidence of these deaths.[404] In the current era of heart failure management, patients survive ventricular arrhythmias and acute exacerbations more often. They then continue to decline until they die of advanced heart failure and end-organ damage.[405]

Patients with Normal Ejection Fraction

Much of the information used to examine the disease course in patients with heart failure is based on data from patients with systolic heart failure. The available evidence on patients with normal EF indicates their disease course is marked by frequent and repeated hospitalizations. These patients experience a symptom burden similar to that of patients with systolic heart failure, and more recent data suggest their mortality is similar.[382,406-408] Causes of death in this population remain predominantly cardiovascular, with 60% of deaths over a 5-year period attributed to sudden death, heart failure, MI, or stroke.[409]

Cardiac Transplantation and Left Ventricular Assist Device

The options of heart transplantation and, to a lesser degree, LVAD implantation offer a longer-lasting way out of the heart failure illness trajectory. Although many patients are ineligible

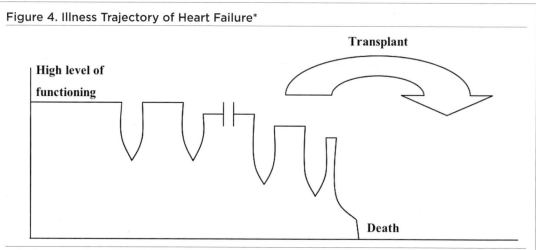

Figure 4. Illness Trajectory of Heart Failure*

Transplant

High level of functioning

Death

The time interval between exacerbations becomes shorter over time and overall functional status diminishes. Heart transplantation offers patients a way off the illness trajectory curve.

for a heart transplant and the number of available organs is limited, the possibility of receiving a transplant and being "cured" of heart failure remains a beacon of hope for many patients and allows them to postpone EOL discussions. Moreover, patients who are incligible for a transplant now can be offered LVAD as destination therapy. Among patients who receive cardiac transplantation, 85% to 90% survive the first year. Roughly 50% of patients with a transplant are alive at year 10, and some patients survive for up to 20 years without needing retransplantation. In an RCT of destination LVAD, patients who had received an LVAD survived 2 years, and patients who had received optimal medical management (OMM) survived for 1 year. The patients who had LVAD implantation also reported better QOL.[410] A more recent study compared the older pulsatile-flow technology with continuous flow, which has the advantage of being smaller, quieter, and more durable.[411] The continuous flow device was associated with improvements in the primary outcome of survival free from a disabling stroke or reoperation for repair or device replacement (46% vs 11%) and improvements in actuarial 2-year survival (58% vs 25%) compared with pulsatile flow, respectively. Taken together, current evidence suggests end-stage heart failure patients eligible for an LVAD have an average 6-month survival with optimal medical management, 12-month survival with a pulsatile LVAD, and 2-year survival with a continuous flow LVAD.[412] Of note, QOL and functional capacity do not vary between pulsatile and continuous LVAD, with the 6-minute walk time almost doubling in both groups after device placement. Given the advancements in technology for patients with an LVAD, survival for destination patients is likely to continue to improve.

Heart Failure Therapies

During the last 10 years the number of heart failure therapies has increased tremendously. A variety of medical and interventional or surgical therapies have been shown to improve both QOL and survival for patients with heart failure. Therapies for heart failure are designed primarily to alleviate the circulatory congestion that leads to many of the symptoms of heart failure that decrease survival and QOL.[413] Because most patients studied in clinical trials of heart failure therapy have systolic heart failure, the information that follows pertains only to those patients unless otherwise indicated.

Medical Therapies

The mainstay of current oral therapy for heart failure includes ACE inhibitors, beta blockers, and diuretics.[414] African Americans also benefit from the addition of hydralazine and nitrates in NYHA class III and IV heart failure after optimization with the aforementioned agents.[383] Spironolactone, administered for further inhibition of the renin-angiotensin-aldosterone system, also is indicated for patients with NYHA Class III and IV symptoms. RCTs have shown that all of these therapies improve survival and QOL. For a detailed summary of these medications, see **Table 12**.[382,383,415]

Patients with adequate renal function should receive diuretics to achieve euvolemia, and those taking ACE inhibitors or angiotensin receptor blockers (ARBs) and beta blockers as stable outpatients should have the drugs titrated up to the maximum tolerated dosage. ACE inhibitors can be initiated if tolerated for afterload reduction during acute hospitalization. ACE inhibitors, ARBs, and spironolactone always should be prescribed in conjunction with an adequate diuretic regimen (**Figure 5**). Some patients whose HF is refractory to loop diuretics benefit from the addition of metolazone.[416] Outpatient management of

Table 12. Medical Therapies for Heart Failure

Class	Examples	Route	Indication	Adverse Effects	Comments
Loop diuretics	Furosemide, torsemide, bumetanide	IV, PO	Volume overload	Renal dysfunction, frequent urination, increased thirst	First-line therapy for volume management in combination with fluid restriction
					IV use may be necessary for acute exacerbations.
Thiazide diuretics	Metolazone, hydrochlorothiazide	PO	Volume overload	Renal dysfunction, frequent urination, increased thirst	Can be added to a loop diuretic for patients not responding to loop diuretic alone
Aldosterone blockers	Spironolactone, eplerenone	PO	NYHA Class III or IV HF	Hyperkalemia, renal dysfunction	Improves survival and functioning in patients with NYHA Class III or IV HF only; patients, especially those with renal insufficiency, should be monitored closely for hyperkalemia; should be administered only in conjunction with loop diuretics.
ACE inhibitors	Captopril, enalapril, lisinopril, ramipril	PO	ACC/AHA stages B-D HF	Hyperkalemia, renal dysfunction, hypotension, cough, angioedema	First-line therapy for systolic HF; may be added to minimize symptoms in patients with preserved EF; some patients in stage D may not tolerate secondary to adverse effects of renal dysfunction, hyperkalemia, and hypotension.
Angiotensin receptor blockers	Candesartan, losartan, valsartan	PO	Patients in ACC/AHA HF stages B-D refractory to ACE inhibitors because of cough or angioedema	Hyperkalemia, renal dysfunction, hypotension	Use of these agents in addition to ACE inhibitors is not indicated.
Beta blockers	Carvedilol, metoprolol	PO	ACC/AHA HF stages B-D	Fatigue, hypotension, depressed mood	First-line therapy for systolic HF; may be added to minimize symptoms in patients with preserved EF; some patients in stage D may not tolerate secondary to adverse effects
Cardiac glycosides	Digoxin	IV, PO	HF that is symptomatic despite administration of first-line therapies	Cardiac arrhythmias, nausea and vomiting, visual hallucinations, delirium	Beta blockers have replaced digoxin for rate control in patients with HF who have atrial fibrillation; monitor for toxicity for elderly patients and for patients with renal insufficiency.

continued

Table 12. Medical Therapies for Heart Failure *continued*

Class	Examples	Route	Indication	Adverse Effects	Comments
IV inotropes	Dobutamine, milrinone	IV	HF stage D	Increased cardiac arrhythmias, decreased survival rates, infectious complications of indwelling central line	Costly; can improve quality of life, but shortens survival
Natriuretic peptides	Nesiritide	IV	Volume overload refractory to diuretics	Renal dysfunction, hypotension	May worsen long-term outcomes
Nitrates	Isosorbide dinitrate	IV, PO	Volume overload, patients requiring afterload reduction	Headache, hypotension	Patients can develop nitrate tolerance and need a nitrate "holiday."
Other vasodilators	Hydralazine	IV, PO	Volume overload, patients requiring afterload reduction	Hypotension, lupus-like syndrome, flushing, nausea, headache	Data on its beneficial effects with nitrates predominantly in African-American populations

ACE, angiotensin converting enzyme; HF, heart failure; IV, intravenous; NYHA, New York Heart Association; PO, by mouth.

these medications requires close monitoring of daily weight and frequent evaluation of serum potassium and creatinine levels, especially during periods when doses of diuretics, ACE inhibitors, ARBs, or spironolactone are being adjusted.[382]

In some cases oral therapies alone are insufficient to achieve euvolemia and improve symptoms of congestion. Patients in these situations often require hospitalization and administration of IV diuretics and possibly IV inotropes to achieve euvolemia before initiating a stable oral diuretic regimen. Some patients' conditions have been managed successfully at home using subcutaneous furosemide infusions.[417] IV nesiritide, a b-type natriuretic peptide, is occasionally helpful for severe dyspnea but has not been shown to extend life, and its use should be limited.[418]

Patients with low cardiac output can experience confusion, lethargy, fatigue, and abdominal discomfort in addition to worsening end-organ function. The appropriate role of inotropic infusions for these patients remains unclear. Data on improved QOL are mixed, and mortality (on either dobutamine or milrinone) may be increased.[415,419] As one expert in the field put it

Reluctance to confront the impending end of life may lead to the complex prescription of home inotropic infusions, requiring indwelling central catheters with high infection risks, and precious community nursing resources. This approach complicates the end of life.[413]

For some patients, it is not possible to discontinue IV inotropes in the hospital because of symptom recurrence or worsening end-organ function. Options for these patients include referral for cardiac transplantation, LVAD, or chronic outpatient inotropes infusion. Patients who remain on chronic IV inotropes and who do not receive LVAD or cardiac transplantation experience an improved QOL compared with similar patients, but they have a decreased rate of survival even with resynchronization therapy.[415,420]

It is important to remember that some drug classes can exacerbate heart failure syndrome and should be avoided; in-depth discussions should occur before initiation. Calcium channel blockers, with the exception of vasoselectives, are associated with an increased risk of cardiovascular events. Also, NSAIDs promote sodium retention and peripheral vasoconstriction, which can worsen heart failure symptoms.

Invasive Therapies

A number of invasive therapies have been developed for heart failure that can improve survival and QOL in select patients. They include ICDs, CRTs, destination LVADs, and cardiac transplantation. Stem cell transplants into the myocardium may soon become available.[421] These therapies are described in **Table 13**. Invasive therapies can alter the illness trajectory as noted previously and also influence QOL.[422] Because of their impact on mode of death and the significant burden associated with invasive therapies (see Table 8), a decision to undergo any of these procedures should be carefully considered. In-depth discussion about this decision is an appropriate indication for referral to a palliative care specialist.

In addition to treating volume overload, a major goal of therapy for patients with normal EF is to control hypertension. These patients also benefit from control of tachycardia because a rapid heart rate reduces the time available for adequate ventricular filling. For this reason, beta-blockers, digoxin, and sometimes calcium channel blockers can provide symptomatic relief for these patients. Patients with atrial fibrillation also may benefit from therapies that restore sinus rhythm.[382]

Figure 5. Flowchart for Adding Therapies for Patients with Heart Failure with Low Ejection Fraction

Symptomatic HF with volume overload (NYHA Class II-IV)

Oral loop diuretics

or

IV loop diuretics and/or metolazone for patients refractory to oral loop diuretics

↓

Symptomatic HF with euvolemia (NYHA Class II-IV)

Titrate ACE inhibitor and betablocker to highest dose tolerated

ARB in patients intolerant to ACE inhibitors

↓

Persistant HF symptoms (NYHA Class III-IV)

Spironolactone

Cardiac resynchronization therapy for patients with QRS > 120 milliseconds

↓

Intractable symptoms

LVAD

Cardiac transplantation

IV Inotropes

HF indicates heart failure; NYHA, New York Heart Association; IV, intravenous; ARB, angiotensin receptor blocker; ACE, angiotensin converting enzyme; LVAD, left ventricular assist device

Table 13. Invasive Therapies for Heart Failure[382,423]

Therapy and Definition	Indication	Benefits	Burdens	Notes
ICD—An implanted device that senses potentially fatal heart rhythms such as ventricular tachycardia and ventricular fibrillation and automatically defibrillates the heart to restore sinus rhythm	EF < 35% with expectation of survival > 1 year	Survival	Pain and psychological trauma from ICD firing, including PTSD and inappropriate firing; surgery- and device-related complications, including lead displacement, infection, pocket erosion, pneumothorax; no definitive improvement in QOL or function; may increase heart failure hospitalizations.	ACC/AHA recommend these devices should not be placed in patients who have a prognosis of 1 year or less or do not maintain good functional capacity; devices most commonly placed in patients older than age 70, a population not well represented in published trials.
CRT—A pacemaker with traditional right-ventricular apical pacing, plus a lead pacing the lateral wall of the LV, causing the right and left ventricles to beat in synchrony	NYHA Class III or IV (ambulatory) HF with EF < 35% and QRS duration > 120 ms	Overall improved survival when combined with an ICD; improved symptoms, exercise capacity, and QOL; decreased hospitalizations	Surgery- and device-related complications, including lead displacement, infection, pocket erosion, pneumothorax, diaphragmatic pacing	Among patients, 20%-30% show no clinical response; mortality benefit emerged by 3 months of therapy; CRT device often is coupled with an ICD.
LVAD—An implanted device that channels blood from the left ventricle through a mechanical pump, ejecting blood into the aorta	1. Bridge to transplantation: Need to mechanically support patients to transplantation when condition likely will not allow survival of the waiting period 2. Destination therapy: Ineligible for transplantation, with survival from systolic HF < 1 year	Overall improved survival, exercise capacity, and QOL for destination therapy compared with optimal medical therapy	Bleeding, infection, thromboembolic events, difficult decisions regarding withdrawal of the device when therapeutic goals are no longer likely, death or permanent disability from surgery	Developed as a bridge therapy to cardiac transplantation, now FDA-approved for destination therapy; in early trials all patients died after 2 years of therapy, but survival is likely to be longer because of advancements in newly developed pumps.
Cardiac transplantation	NYHA Class IV HF refractory/intolerant to optimal medical therapy; refractory angina; or ventricular arrhythmias	Overall improved survival and QOL	Significant first-year mortality, need for lifelong immunosuppressive drugs (and ability to tolerate their side effects), uncertainty involved in waiting	Fewer than 2,500 patients each year receive transplantation because of lack of available organs. Fifty percent of patients are alive 10 years after transplantation, and some survive for 20 years.

ACC/AHA, American College of Cardiology/American Heart Association; CRT, cardiac resynchronization therapy; EF, ejection fraction; HF, heart failure; ICD, implantable cardioverter defibrillator; LV, left ventricle; LVAD, left ventricular assist device; NYHA, New York Heart Association; PTSD, posttraumatic stress disorder; QOL, quality of life.

Paul's Case Continues

After a thorough evaluation, Paul's care team deemed he was not a candidate for cardiac transplantation or LVAD placement due to his morbid obesity. He became more debilitated from his illness and was no longer able to work. Paul eventually moved in with his elderly parents because he was unable to afford his apartment. He also experienced increasing difficulty with activities such as grocery shopping, cleaning, doing laundry, and preparing his meals.

Paul was admitted to the hospital for the third time in 2 months due to worsening dyspnea with minimal activity. A palliative medicine consultant was called to help him manage his anxiety. During the interview, Paul expressed his wish to get better but said that fluid restriction was making him terribly thirsty. He said he didn't think he could stand living with such extreme thirst. He also said he was aware that his heart had become worse, but he was certain that he would be able to get better and go home. He said he was not ready to give up and that the only way he could cope with the stress of being in the hospital would be to take lorazepam. On further questioning, he admitted to having pain in his legs related to "swelling."

At the time of physical examination, Paul had pressured speech and psychomotor agitation. He shifted positions in his bed frequently and maintained poor eye contact. He had 3-plus pitting edema of the lower extremities and a massive amount of ascites. On review of his medical record he was found to be taking lorazepam, 1 mg IV every 4 to 6 hours throughout the day. The palliative care team recommended that he start on escitalopram, 10 mg at bedtime for his anxiety, and clonazepam, 0.5 mg three times a day. The lorazepam was discontinued. An order also was placed for oxycodone, 5 mg every 4 hours as needed for his leg pain. A visit with the palliative care psychologist was scheduled for counseling on relaxation techniques to help manage the anxiety related to his thirst.

The following day the nursing staff reported that Paul was sleeping all day and was difficult to rouse. He had received three doses of clonazepam since the previous visit and one dose of oxycodone in the morning. The dosage of clonazepam was decreased to 0.5 mg twice a day, and the dosage of oxycodone was reduced to 2.5 mg as needed. Paul became more alert and his pain was better controlled. He was discharged several days later with a plan to continue outpatient psychotherapy for his anxiety.

Question Five

According to RCT data, what is Paul's 1-year mortality?

A. Less than 5%

B. 5% to 10%

C. 10% to 15%

D. 25%

Correct Response and Analysis

The correct answer is C. According to NYHA classification, 1-year mortality is estimated as 7% for Class II, 13% for Class III, and 20% to 52% for Class IV patients. Paul had NYHA Class III heart failure symptoms at the time of hospital admission (symptoms with minimal activity), which meant that his 1-year mortality, according to RCT data, was 13%.

Question Six

Which of the following statements is true regarding medication management for Paul's symptoms?

A. No dosage adjustment is necessary when initiating long-acting benzodiazepines for patients with heart failure.

B. It is rare for patients with heart failure to become oversedated from opioids.

C. An appropriate starting dosage of an opioid for an opioid-naïve patient with heart failure would be roughly half of the usual starting dosage.

D. His pain and sedation would be better managed through discontinuation of oxycodone and adding ibuprofen, 600 mg by mouth every 8 hours.

Correct Response and Analysis

The correct answer is C. Sedating medications such as opioids or benzodiazepines should be administered at roughly half the usual starting dosage to patients who are naïve to these agents. Long-acting benzodiazepines have a decreased clearance in patients with heart failure, and the dosing interval should be extended. NSAIDs are generally contraindicated in patients with heart failure due to risk for sodium and water retention and adverse effects on kidney function.

Continued on page 74

Advance Care Planning

Prognosis in Heart Failure

When discussing advance care planning with patients and families, it is important to understand the patients' prognosis. Determining an exact prognosis can be difficult for many patients referred for palliative care, and physicians tend to overestimate patient prognosis.[424] The difficulties in describing and predicting the disease course for patients with heart failure are discussed in the Disease Trajectory and Management section. Because of the episodic nature of heart failure and the different ways in which patients die from it, prognostication for patients with heart failure remains challenging. The information that exists about prognosis in heart failure comes from two major sources: RCTs of therapies for heart failure and large community databases. The strengths and weaknesses of these data sources are discussed below.

Extensive studies on therapy for systolic heart failure have been conducted, and many of these studies indicate death as a primary outcome. Clinical characteristics of patients enrolled in the studies are carefully described. For these reasons, such studies are good sources of information on actual mortality rates for specific types of patients. Because almost all of these studies involved therapies for systolic heart failure, it is difficult to generalize their data to patients with normal EF. Moreover, patients enrolled in these trials are carefully selected and often are excluded if they have other comorbid illnesses. In general, they are healthier than the general population. They are also much more likely to adhere to optimal medical therapy. For these reasons, data from these studies tend to underestimate mortality rates. A large review of these data outlined 1-year mortality estimates, categorized according to NYHA classification, as 7% for Class II patients, 13% for Class III patients, and 20% to 52% for Class IV patients.[425]

The data obtained from large community databases have the advantage of inclusion of patients with all types of heart failure who are on real-life therapies. For this reason, they can be generalized to the community of patients with heart failure. However, the data are not class specific, and patient characteristics are not well defined. As a result, it is difficult to find specific estimates to apply to a given patient. Community data from two large databases of outpatients with cardiovascular disease provide 1-year heart failure mortality estimates of 17% and 10-year mortality estimates ranging between 38% and 77%.[425]

A number of prognostic models have been developed in an effort to better describe prognosis in heart failure. Earlier models were based on patients in the hospital, which makes them difficult to use when assessing patients in an outpatient setting. Many of the models developed for outpatients required data that are not routinely available, such as right-heart catheterization or cardiopulmonary exercise testing. One published model used only easily obtainable laboratory data from outpatients.[426] The authors discovered the following independent risk factors that contribute to a worse prognosis:

- more severe NYHA classification
- ischemic etiology
- low EF
- low systolic blood pressure
- low serum sodium.

Because the model uses a high number of both continuous and categorical variables, it is too complex to allow manual calculation of prognosis. For this reason, a useful online calculator has been made available at http://depts.washington.edu/shfm (Accessed January 8, 2012). The calculator provides 1-, 2-, and 5-year mortality estimates and survival curves and estimates of the impact of specific heart-failure therapies on survival.[426] It is important to note that most of the patients upon which the model was based, developed, and validated had systolic heart failure, which made data difficult to generalize to patients with normal EF. Also, because the model was based on stable outpatients, when applying it to patients in the hospital it is best to use NYHA symptoms and laboratory values from the most recent stable outpatient visit.

Information about prognosis for patients with very advanced heart failure in an era of more sophisticated heart-failure therapies is available from several recent studies. The Randomized Evaluation of Mechanical Assistance for the Treatment of Congestive Heart Failure study was an RCT of destination LVAD versus OMM for patients with inotrope-dependent Class III or IV heart failure. Sixty-one patients were enrolled in the OMM arm of the study. Their mortality

was 50% at 6 months, 75% at 12 months, and almost 100% at 2 years. The Continuous Outpatient Support with Inotropes study followed 36 patients on home inotropic support. Mortality for these patients was 60% at 6 months and 94% at 1 year. Multiple RCTs comparing CRT with OMM have been published.[423,427] In the Comparison of Medical Therapy, Pacing, and Defibrillation in Heart Failure study, 308 patients with Class III or IV heart failure and EF lower than 35% were enrolled in the OMM arm. Twenty-five percent of these patients died during the 12-month study period.[428] These studies are summarized in **Table 14**.[428-430]

Communication

Effective communication between patients and clinicians is a cornerstone of good palliative care. Patients with heart failure have strong preferences about what is most important for their care. In two studies, patients were allowed to choose between shorter survival time and improvement in QOL versus longer survival time at their current QOL. Both studies revealed strong polarity of preference in either direction, with a large group of patients choosing QOL over survival and another group choosing prolonged survival over improvement in their QOL.[431,432]

Treating physicians often are not aware of these strong patient preferences. In a SUPPORT study, physicians and their patients were independently interviewed about resuscitation preferences. Twenty-three percent of patients did not want to be resuscitated, but only 25% of those patients had accurately relayed this information to their physicians.[433] Another study found that only 5% of patients hospitalized for heart failure had DNAR orders recorded in their charts.[434] In another study, caregivers of patients who died from heart failure were interviewed. They found that as many as 50% of patients were aware they were dying, and 80% of them came to that

Table 14. Mortality for Patients with Advanced Heart Failure Receiving Optimal Medical Management Trials[428-430]

Study Name	Study Description	Enrollment Period	Patient Characteristics	1-Year Mortality	Median Survival
Randomized Evaluation of Mechanical Assistance for the Treatment of Congestive Heart Failure	RCT of LVAD vs OMM	1998-2001	NYHA Class III and inotropes or balloon-pump dependence, or NYHA Class IV	75%	150 days
Continuous Outpatient Support Study	Prospective observational study of chronic outpatient inotropes	1993-2002	ACC/AHA stage D outpatients on chronic IV inotropes plus other OMM	94%	3.4 months
Comparison of Medical Therapy, Pacing, and Defibrillation in Heart Failure	RCT of CRT vs OMM	2000-2002	NYHA Class III or IV with EF < 35%	25%	Not applicable

CRT, cardiac resynchronization therapy; EF, ejection fraction; IV, intravenous; LVAD, left ventricular assistive device; NYHA, New York Heart Association; OMM, optimal medical management; RCT, randomized controlled trial.

realization on their own.[435] These findings confirm that patients with heart failure have strong preferences regarding their care and often know death is imminent, yet they still fail to share that information with their physicians. The need for improved communication about goals of care is an important consideration for palliative care clinicians caring for patients with heart failure.[388]

In addition to improving communication about advance directives, early palliative care for heart failure also can help patients and families make complex decisions surrounding invasive and potentially disease-altering therapies such as ICD, CRT, LVAD,[436] or transplantation. Such interventions may be offered shortly after diagnosis, especially for patients who develop cardiogenic shock at first presentation of CHF. Moreover, many patients who receive invasive therapies such as ICDs do not have appropriate discussions with their caregivers and physicians about discontinuing their use when goals change or the disease progresses. One study in which family members of patients with an ICD who died of advanced heart failure were interviewed found that 45% of patients who had a standing DNAR order had not had their devices deactivated. Thirty percent of these patients experienced a shock during their last month of life, and 8% experienced a shock during their final minutes of life.[437] In light of these findings it is increasingly important for palliative care specialists to help facilitate communication about advance directives.

For a more detailed discussion of communication in palliative care, see *UNIPAC 5*.

Paul's Case Continues

One week later Paul presented to the ED with severe shortness of breath and nausea. He was found to be hypotensive and in acute renal failure. His weight had increased by 20 pounds since his discharge, and he admitted that he had not been able to adhere to his fluid-restriction or diuretic regimens. To maintain blood pressure, he was started on IV inotropic support with dobutamine. With this therapy, his nausea and shortness of breath improved. He began to urinate and his renal function improved modestly. However, whenever the cardiology team attempted to wean him off the dobutamine, his nausea returned and his renal function worsened.

The palliative care team was asked to address goals of care. Paul reported that although his anxiety had decreased, he could no longer stand being in the hospital and could not continue to live with such severe thirst. He stated that he would rather live for a shorter time in a place he loved surrounded by his family. The palliative-care team discussed the option of discharge from the hospital with palliative care and possibly hospice. Paul's extended family supported his decision and made plans to take him to a family home in the mountains that had always been one of his favorite places.

Plans were made for Paul's discharge. Because his nausea and dyspnea were much better on dobutamine, the palliative care team decided it should be continued for palliation. Paul's medications were reviewed and he was discharged on IV dobutamine. His diuretics were continued but at less frequent dosing intervals, and he was allowed to drink more than 2 L of fluids per day. He was scheduled to receive palliative home nursing because hospice in his area was unable to provide continuous IV dobutamine. The palliative care team spoke to Paul about his ICD and explained that it likely would not prolong his life and could also prevent his death

from being peaceful. He agreed to have his ICD deactivated before discharge.

Question Seven

Which of the following should be considered when discussing deactivation of Paul's ICD?

A. Patients who wish for a peaceful death should be informed that active ICDs may fire at their time of death, which could be traumatic.

B. ICDs are unlikely to work if they fire while a patient is imminently dying.

C. The most definitive way to deactivate an ICD is to have the device reprogrammed.

D. A and C

E. A, B, and C

Correct Response and Analysis

The correct response is E. Discussions about deactivating ICDs should focus on the patient's or surrogate's goals of care, keeping in mind the end-stage nature of the disease and close proximity to death. ICDs may fire when death is near, leading to unnecessary discomfort in a dying patient. Definitive deactivation of an ICD should be conducted by an electrophysiologist who can reprogram the device not to fire. If this is not possible, a magnet may be placed over the device to prevent it from sensing an abnormal rhythm, however this "magnet mode" may not be active in certain devices.

Question Eight

Which of the following is true regarding palliative medicine and hospice care for Paul?

A. Many therapies for CHF are no longer effective when patients are end stage; consequently, his oral medications should be discontinued.

B. The median length of stay for heart failure patients in hospice is 60 days.

C. Home inotropic support is likely to improve survival.

D. Paul's parents are at risk for depressive symptoms, stress, and increased caregiver burden.

Correct Response and Analysis

The correct response is D. A number of studies have documented that caregivers of people with heart failure report high stress, burden, depression, and poor overall health. Variables associated with a diminished caregiver QOL include caring for a younger patient, larger caregiver burden, and decreased caregiver sense of control. Because many oral therapies such as diuretics and ACE inhibitors help control symptoms, they should be continued throughout the disease course until burdens outweigh the expected benefits. The challenges surrounding early palliative care referral and hospice enrollment for people with heart failure involve prognostication, advance care planning, and widespread views that heart failure is not a life-limiting condition. As a result, the median length of stay in hospice is fairly short at around 10 days. Although home inotropic support may improve symptoms and QOL, no data suggest it can improve survival. Such support is associated with high cost and may increase the incidence of cardiac arrhythmias and line infections. Goals, burdens, and cost of care should be carefully considered before offering a patient home inotropic support.

Heart failure is an illness that often is marked by exacerbations alternating with periods of stability. The mode of death for patients with heart failure is variable.[405] Some patients die suddenly from ventricular arrhythmias, some fail to recover from an acute exacerbation, and some eventually die of advanced disease and end-organ failure. When providing palliative care to these patients during the final days or hours of their lives, it is important to understand how death might occur, the symptoms these patients might experience, and when withdrawal of certain therapies might be appropriate.

Continued on page 82

Symptom Management

Patients with heart failure experience significant symptoms during the course of their disease that can profoundly affect their QOL. When treating patients with heart failure with potentially sedating drugs such as opioids, benzodiazepines, anticonvulsants, and sedating antidepressants and antipsychotics, it is important to understand that these patients often have impaired clearance of medications and metabolites because of a high frequency of impaired renal function or impaired hepatic function. In addition, patients with low cardiac output can experience confusion and sedation from cerebral hypoperfusion alone without the addition of sedating medications. For these reasons, it is best practice to start these drugs at a low dosage, usually half of what generally would be prescribed to an otherwise healthy person with normal renal function. Care should be taken to spread out dosing intervals for long-acting medications, such as sustained-release opioids and long-acting benzodiazepines.

Dyspnea

A significant number of patients with advanced heart failure experience dyspnea as a prominent symptom. The primary treatment for dyspnea in patients with heart failure involves first attempting to treat volume overload with cardiac medications. For patients in the final stages of illness this may not be possible. For such patients, it is appropriate to initiate opioid treatment for dyspnea.[438] For outpatients or inpatients who are not in acute respiratory failure, low-dose oral morphine or oxycodone often are helpful if initially administered on an as-needed basis. If patients improve and are taking a stable amount of drug, sustained-release formulations can be prescribed at twice-daily dosing intervals. For patients in the inpatient setting who are acutely dying of respiratory failure, bolus IV opioids are appropriate, as are concentrated sublingual (SL) opioids for patients in the home hospice setting.

In addition, some patients experience anxiety as a result of their dyspnea and may benefit from anxiolytic therapy with a low-dose benzodiazepine or atypical antipsychotic. Other patients may benefit from therapies such as medical air or supplemental oxygen.[439] A number of nonpharmacologic methods also have been shown to be effective, including facial cooling, improved air circulation with a fan, or neuromuscular electrical stimulation.[283]

For more detailed discussion about palliative therapies for dyspnea, see the section on Dyspnea and *UNIPAC 4*.

Pain

Patients with heart failure commonly experience pain.[440] Etiologies for pain in these patients are many and often are related to other comorbid illnesses rather than to heart failure itself. For this reason, a careful history and physical examination are important to diagnose the specific etiology for pain and its appropriate treatment. For example, a patient with pain from ischemia resulting from vascular disease would benefit from an opioid, but a patient with pain from diabetic neuropathy would benefit from therapies targeted to neuropathic pain such as antidepressants or anticonvulsants.[389] Again, exercise caution by starting with low dosages and using broad dosing intervals. NSAIDs generally are contraindicated in heart failure because of their effects on kidney function and sodium and fluid retention, which can worsen heart failure and increase hospitalization rates. Alternative considerations may include thermal modalities (heat and cold), topical agents (creams and balms), and joint injections with a steroid and local anesthetic for localized pain.

For detailed information on therapies for specific pain syndromes and dosing information, see *UNIPAC 3*.

Anxiety and Depression

Nearly 50% of patients with advanced heart failure experience psychiatric symptoms of anxiety and depression that can be disabling. Untreated anxiety and depression can aggravate other symptoms such as pain and dyspnea, and untreated depression and insomnia can contribute to fatigue.

Patients with depression can be treated with cognitive behavioral psychotherapy, SSRIs, selective serotonin/norepinephrine reuptake inhibitors (SNRIs), mirtazapine, and bupropion.[441] SNRIs should be used carefully for patients with hypertension or atrial fibrillation because they can elevate blood pressure and aggravate tachycardia. Mirtazapine can be helpful for patients with insomnia or anorexia as components of their depression, but it should be started slowly because of oversedation risk. Tricyclic antidepressants including nortriptyline or desipramine also may be considered but can adversely affect the conduction system, leading to changes in the QT interval. Although psychostimulants are generally avoided for patients with heart disease because of risk for ventricular arrhythmias, they can sometimes be started at low dosages for select patients with no prior history of arrhythmia. No data currently exist to support the safety of one psychostimulant over another for this population. When using these agents for patients with heart failure, it is best to start the medication only after consultation with the patient's cardiologist and to initiate therapy in the hospital with the patient on telemetry. In addition, patients with heart failure can benefit from psychotherapy alone or in combination with medical therapy.

The first-line treatment for anxiety in heart failure is medical therapy in conjunction with cognitive behavioral therapy for relaxation training. Medical therapy should consist of an antidepressant such as an SSRI. Because antidepressants can take several weeks to reach therapeutic efficacy, short-term relief can be provided by administering a low-dose benzodiazepine such as clonazepam or an atypical antipsychotic such as olanzapine or quetiapine. Quetiapine, when given at low doses of 12.5 mg at bedtime, can be helpful for patients who have insomnia as a component of their anxiety. This drug may be preferable to sedative-hypnotic sleep aids that can accumulate and cause morning drug hangover.

Fatigue

Fatigue is a prominent symptom for patients with heart failure. Most often it is directly related to heart failure itself or to beta blocker therapy. However, patients who say they have fatigue should be carefully evaluated for other treatable causes. Patients with heart failure and anemia did not see improvements in their exercise tolerance or their QOL when treated with darbepoetin alpha.[442] In a small series, testosterone supplementation appeared to increase strength and functional capacity in both men and women with advanced heart failure.[443]

Sleep-disordered breathing is common in patients with heart failure and can cause significant fatigue. Patients with symptoms of nonrestorative sleep or daytime somnolence should be referred for evaluation for and possible treatment of sleep apnea. Insomnia experienced as a part of depression, anxiety, or situational factors should be treated.

Patients with profound fatigue not caused by a comorbid condition likely are experiencing this symptom as a result of their advanced disease. These patients sometimes are treated with IV inotropes, but there is questionable evidence related to associated benefits, high costs, and decreased survival.[382,413,415] Psychostimulants can be used with caution for select patients.

Nausea

Patients with low cardiac output, abdominal ascites, or both may experience nausea as a prominent symptom of decompensated heart failure. These patients should be treated for volume overload with diuretics and may require the addition of inotropic support if diuretics alone do not relieve their symptoms. Even when undergoing therapy for volume overload or in situations in which volume overload is no longer aggressively managed, patients may benefit from antiemetics such as ondansetron, haloperidol, metoclopramide, or prochlorperazine. Sedating agents such as prochlorperazine should be started at a lower dosage initially and titrated upward as tolerated.

End-Stage Issues

Mode of Death

Hospitalized patients with heart failure who fail to recover from an acute exacerbation may die of respiratory failure as a result of refractory volume overload and pulmonary edema. They might also fail to recover enough cardiac output to maintain adequate blood pressure. Dyspnea from respiratory failure should be managed with IV, subcutaneous (SC), or SL administration of opioids given at 15- to 30-minute intervals and titrated upward if necessary to relieve air hunger and respiratory distress. Terminal agitation can be managed with IV or SL haloperidol on an as-needed basis. Patients who experience anxiety or restlessness sometimes benefit from IV or SL administration of a benzodiazepine.

For patients who are not dying of an acute exacerbation but rather from progression to end-stage organ failure, acute respiratory distress is much less common. These patients gradually experience loss of consciousness because of uremia and poor cerebral perfusion. The dyspnea they experience often is more chronic than acute. Hyponatremia and acute chronic renal insufficiency is common.[444] Treatment for these patients should focus on alleviating any pain that may be present, continuing to manage chronic dyspnea, and treating terminal agitation with antipsychotics.

Withdrawing Life-Prolonging Therapies

Invasive therapies for heart failure such as ICDs or destination LVAD can improve survival for patients and sometimes improve their QOL. However, when a patient reaches a point in his or her illness when therapies no longer provide these benefits or when death is imminent, it is important to discuss with the patient or the patient's family or surrogate how and when these therapies might be withdrawn. Ideally, the circumstances under which a therapy might be withdrawn is something that is discussed before its initiation,[445] and clear advance directives should be in place for surrogates. The Heart Rhythm Society has published a consensus statement that incorporates input from several stakeholders including the American Academy of Hospice and Palliative Medicine regarding the management of ICDs and CRT in patients nearing EOL.[446] These guidelines include a detailed discussion of the legal, ethical, and religious aspects that surround device deactivation, along with communication techniques to facilitate a "goals of care" conversation. The ACC/AHA continues to recommend that physicians give patients with stage D heart failure information about deactivation of their ICDs.[382] In practice, this often is not the case.[447] Palliative care clinicians often help guide these decisions during the final stage of illness.

When discussing deactivation of an ICD, it is important to learn from the patient or surrogate what the patient's goals are while being mindful of the fact that he or she is reaching the end stage of the disease and that death may be imminent. Patients who want their death to be peaceful should be told that if their ICD were to remain active, the device may fire at the time of their death, which could be traumatic for them. It is also important to inform them that if the device were to fire, it likely would not save their life in very advanced disease. After learning this information, most patients and families agree to have the device deactivated. The most definitive way to deactivate an ICD is for an electrophysiologist or a representative from the company that inserted the device to reprogram the device. This is not an invasive procedure and takes only a few moments. In most cases, a magnet placed over the device will prevent it from sensing an abnormal rhythm. However, in some instances this "magnet mode" may not be active in the device, and placing a magnet over it may not prevent it from sensing a ventricular arrhythmia and firing. For this reason, using a magnet to deactivate the device should be a last resort.

Patients receiving circulatory support from an LVAD face a complex situation at EOL. These patients often survive until the time their device is turned off. Because death is often immediate after withdrawal of the device, the decision can be stressful for patients and families. However, when a patient's goals no longer are realized by continuing this support, it is appropriate to withdraw it.[448] Withdrawal of an LVAD generally takes place in a hospital, where LVAD technicians can turn down the flow on the pumps and turn off the device. After the device is withdrawn, patients often develop acute pulmonary edema and circulatory collapse. Managing their symptoms at the time the device is withdrawn should be similar to the care given to patients at the time of a terminal wean from full ventilatory support. Patients should be premedicated with IV opioids and benzodiazepines before the device is withdrawn, and additional doses should be readily available in the event the patient develops evidence of pain or respiratory distress. One center reported that the most common reasons cited for withdrawing LVAD support included declining functional ability, worsening and/or new comorbidities, and limited family interaction due to declining cognition. When the pump was deactivated, all patients became unconscious, and death followed within 20 minutes.[449]

Psychological and Spiritual Care
The final phase of illness can be difficult for both patients and those who care for them. Because of the episodic nature of heart failure, many patients and families are well prepared in advance of the patient's death. The need to make decisions about withdrawing therapies can cause additional emotional and spiritual distress. These patients and their families should be given ample psychological and spiritual support. For more details on providing support and addressing spiritual pain, see *UNIPAC 2*.

Palliative Care and Hospice

Patients with advanced heart failure may benefit from palliative home care or hospice.[405] However, many barriers exist that prevent or delay the delivery of palliative care for these patients. Difficulty determining when and how death might occur makes advance care planning challenging. The multitude of medical and surgical therapies for heart failure provide potential alternative courses of therapy for patients; often these therapies become the focus of care and de-emphasize the need for EOL care. The fact that CHF is a life-limiting condition is still not widely accepted among patients or physicians.[240,450]

After heart failure patients are referred to hospice, the care they require may differ from care rendered to other hospice patients. Many active therapies for heart failure also improve QOL and should not necessarily be discontinued when a patient enters hospice. In addition, many patients can feel significantly better after a short stay in the hospital for management of volume overload. The timing of referral and which therapies to continue at home should be assessed carefully and fully discussed.

Timing of Referral
Traditional models of palliative care, based on treatment for patients with cancer, recommended little or no role for palliative care at the time of diagnosis, advising that palliative care should assume increasing prominence as a disease progresses. Curative therapies often are discontinued toward the end of a patient's life. Some have proposed a different model for patients with heart failure, one in which palliative care would have a more active role at the time of diagnosis, with some active or curative therapies continuing until the time of death (**Figure 6**). At the time of diagnosis, palliative care would consist primarily of facilitating communication about decisions of

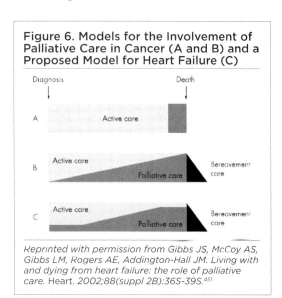

Figure 6. Models for the Involvement of Palliative Care in Cancer (A and B) and a Proposed Model for Heart Failure (C)

Reprinted with permission from Gibbs JS, McCoy AS, Gibbs LM, Rogers AE, Addington-Hall JM. Living with and dying from heart failure: the role of palliative care. Heart. 2002;88(suppl 2B):36S-39S.[451]

whether to pursue invasive therapies such as ICD, LVAD, or transplantation. As in the cancer model, the role for palliative care would become increasingly prominent as the disease progresses, but some active heart-failure therapies would continue until the time of death, even for patients for whom the goal of care is not prolonged survival.[451]

Hospice Care

Although more people in the United States die of heart disease than of all cancers combined,[452] more hospice admissions and opioid prescriptions are for patients with cancer.[453] In 2009, 40.1% of all US hospice patients died of cancer while only 11.5% died of heart disease.[454] There are multiple explanations for this apparent discrepancy. First, it is likely that the episodic disease course of heart failure and the difficulties determining prognosis for it play a key role. In addition, the fact that heart failure is a life-limiting condition is still not widely accepted by patients or physicians.[240] Finally, although both cardiologists and palliative care clinicians are beginning to advocate for palliative care and hospice for patients with advanced heart failure,[382,394] there is little hard evidence about the specific needs of patients referred to these services.

The small amount of data that exist on hospice care for heart failure come from a retrospective study of a hospice caring for these patients. These data show that many of these patients were elderly and that their length of stay was fairly short, with the median length of stay at only 10 days.[455] The settings for hospice delivery included home (42%), long-term care facilities (31%), and inpatient hospice units (21%).[455] These patients made use of more traditional hospice comfort medications such as opioids, anxiolytics, antidepressants, and scopolamine. Most of these hospice patients had made use of the hospice interdisciplinary team, including social work, volunteer, and chaplaincy support; most died at home.[455] Another retrospective study of heart failure hospice patients corroborated that a large proportion of patients have a short stay.[456] In fact, the proportion of heart failure patients with a length of stay of 7 or fewer days was similar to that of cancer patients—31.7% versus 30.8% ($P = .08$), respectively. Few patients (19%) were prescribed standard therapy with an ACE inhibitor or ARB and beta blocker.

Determining the timing of hospice enrollment for patients with heart failure also can be challenging. Much of this challenge stems from difficulty predicting prognosis in heart failure. The National Hospice and Palliative Care Organization's 1996 guidelines for heart-failure admission to hospice include the following criteria*:

- presence of symptoms at rest
- optimal medical treatment
- EF < 20%
- unexplained syncope
- resistant ventricular or supraventricular arrythmias.

It is important to note that, based on current medical literature, these guidelines are not predictive of 6- or 12-month prognosis with 50% accuracy.[457] For this reason, it is best practice to make a clinical judgment based on each patient's goals of therapy, their NYHA classification, and any medical comorbidities. In general, patients with NYHA Class III or IV heart failure who wish to forgo frequent hospital admissions, transplant,

*Editor's note. NHPCO recommends that providers research the local coverage determinations (LCDs) that apply to their state by using the Medicare coverage database, which can be found at www.cms.gov/medicare-coverage-database/overview-and-quick-search.aspx (Accessed February 6, 2012). These LCDs will provide information regarding disease-specific factors and prognosis, because the final determination and information about disease appropriateness rests with each hospice Medicare Administrative Contractor (MAC). We include this information here as a starting point for determining a patient's eligibility for hospice services but encourage physicians to refer to their LCDs and MACs for current information (NHPCO, personal communication, January 27, 2012).

~~or LVAD therapy are good candidates for hospice referral.~~

Management of Cardiac Therapies for Palliation

Many active therapies for heart failure also provide relief of symptoms and improve QOL. For this reason, many of these medications should be continued throughout the entire disease course. For example, ACE inhibitors and beta blockers help to improve functional status and contribute to QOL. They should be continued until the burdens of therapy outweigh the benefits. Because patients feel better when they are free of congestion, diuretics and some level of fluid restriction should be continued throughout the disease course. If the burdens of the patient's diuretic regimen are not acceptable to him or her at the prescribed frequency, it may be possible for him or her to benefit from the diuretics at less frequent dosing intervals. Similarly, fluid restriction might be lessened and patients might be allowed more indiscretions. Such strategies allow the clinician and patient to negotiate a balance between the burdens and the benefits of the therapies.

Other active therapies, such as IV or SC diuretics and brief treatment with inotropes, may sometimes return a patient to a desired level of functioning. An open discussion about goals of care is essential. Some patients may elect to revoke their hospice enrollment in favor of continuing these therapies. Sometimes hospices can provide the therapies at home, making postponing or revoking hospice enrollment unnecessary.

Some patients become "dependent" on IV inotropes during a hospital admission. Some patients may feel better on dobutamine or milrinone, but there no evidence that either drug is superior,[419] and there is little convincing evidence that home inotropic support improves QOL. The high cost, complexity, and risk of complications of this therapy, which is known to shorten survival, is difficult to justify. For these reasons, the goals, burdens, and costs of care should be addressed before offering a patient home inotropic support for palliation. Because these patients often experience a higher incidence of ventricular arrhythmias, deactivation of ICDs should be recommended before discharge.

Hospice Enrollment

For enrollment into hospice, a physician is required to certify that a patient has a 6-month prognosis. Given the difficulties of prognostication for heart failure, one must accept that patients who are likely to benefit from hospice enrollment may survive for more than 6 months. Because patients with NYHA Class III or IV heart failure have a high 1-year mortality, it is reasonable to enroll these patients in hospice when QOL becomes more important to them than aggressively pursuing disease-altering therapies such as LVAD or transplantation. Hospice referral is also appropriate when these patients begin to express a desire to forgo frequent hospital admissions. This being said, some hospice patients may benefit from a chest X ray, cardiology consultation, or IV diuretics for treatment of acute exacerbations. In addition, some patients may choose to receive hospice care to improve QOL and, at the same time, hope to receive a heart transplant. As long as these decisions are carefully discussed, advance directives are in place, and the patient does not require frequent hospital admissions, continued care in hospice can remain the most appropriate option.

Role of the Interdisciplinary Team

As with other diagnoses, patients with heart failure benefit most from the care of the entire interdisciplinary team. These benefits support early referral to hospice or palliative care. For more details on the role of the interdisciplinary team, see *UNIPAC 5*.

Paul's Case Concludes

Initially Paul felt well enough at home to enjoy interacting with his family. He gradually improved with the dobutamine but had little appetite and was mostly bedbound. He was able to enjoy several gourmet meals. Two weeks after discharge, Paul's sister called his cardiologist to report that his edema and shortness of breath were worsening and to ask why her brother was being given a medication known to shorten life. She said that Paul also was having impaired cognition and was sleeping for most of the day. The decision was made to transfer Paul to home hospice care and take him off of his dobutamine because it was no longer helpful. Concentrated liquid morphine and lorazepam were available in the home and were given to Paul to treat his shortness of breath and anxiety before withdrawal of the dobutamine. He died peacefully in the presence of his family 1 month later in the family's mountain home.

Caregiver Issues

Patients with heart failure experience loss of functioning relatively early in their disease course. For this reason, family members and other caregivers often play a prominent role in their lives. A number of studies document that caregivers of people with heart failure report high stress, burden, depressive symptoms, and poorer overall health.[458] A number of studies have examined the impact of caring for a patient with heart failure on the caregiver's QOL. One study of 67 patient-spouse pairs found that the overall emotional well-being of caregivers was significantly worse than that of the general population. The study noted three variables predicting diminished caregiver QOL: (a) younger age of patient, (b) larger caregiver burden, and (c) decreased caregiver-perceived control.[459] Another study examined the impact of caring for a patient receiving IV inotropic support in a community setting. This study examined 20 patients and their primary caregivers and measured their mental health scores. Among caregivers, 89% were found to have mental health scores that were lower than their established age norm. Caregivers were proud of the care they were providing but identified negative aspects of their caregiver experience, such as time constraints on their day-to-day lives, costs to their own health, and financial burden.[437] When providing complete hospice and palliative care to patients with heart failure, it is important to recognize the burden of illness on the patient and those involved in caring for the patient. Efforts should be made to help manage financial burdens, maximize the physical health of caregivers, and empower caregivers to have more perceived control.

Reduction of Burden

As discussed previously, family members often are faced with managing financial difficulties related to caring for their loved ones. Hospice and palliative care case managers and social workers can help patients and families navigate the healthcare system and manage these stressors. Moreover, respite care through hospice can give caregivers a reprieve from the day-to-day burden of caring for the patient. Because they alleviate some of the physical suffering brought on by illness, palliative care and hospice personnel can help caregivers feel confident they have done all they can for the patient. Family members often experience stress related to making difficult decisions for their loved ones.[372] Assistance with these decisions and careful advance care planning can help ease the stress of this decision making.

Bereavement Support

Because patients with heart failure often require a great deal of care for long periods, caregivers often find they spend most of their time taking care of the patient. After the patient dies, caregivers often find themselves with nothing left to occupy their time. This, in combination with grief over the loss of their loved one, can be difficult. Bereavement follow-up is a fundamental part of good palliative care and should be provided to caregivers.[460] For more information on bereavement support, see *UNIPAC 5.*

References

1.	Lanctot KL, Herrmann N, Rothenburg L, Eryavec G. Behavioral correlates of GABAergic disruption in Alzheimer's disease. *Int Psychogeriatr.* 2007;19(1):151-158.

2.	Petersen RC, Smith G, Kokmen E, Ivnik RJ, Tangalos EG. Memory function in normal aging. *Neurology.* 1992;42(2):396-401.

3.	Busse A, Angermeyer MC, Riedel-Heller SG. Progression of mild cognitive impairment to dementia: a challenge to current thinking. *Br J Psychiatry.* 2006;189:399-404.

4.	Barker WW, Luis CA, Kashuba A, et al. Relative frequencies of Alzheimer disease, Lewy body, vascular and frontotemporal dementia, and hippocampal sclerosis in the State of Florida Brain Bank. *Alzheimer Dis Assoc Disord.* 2002;16(4):203-212.

5.	Blennow K, de Leon MJ, Zetterberg H. Alzheimer's disease. *Lancet.* 2006;368(9533):387-403.

6.	Morris JC, McKeel DW, Jr., Fulling K, Torack RM, Berg L. Validation of clinical diagnostic criteria for Alzheimer's disease. *Ann Neurol.* 1988;24(1):17-22.

7.	American Psychiatric Association. *Diagnostic and Statistical Manual of Mental Disorders.* 4th ed. Arlington, VA: American Psychiatric Publishing, Inc; 2000.

8.	McKhann G, Drachman D, Folstein M, Katzman R, Price D, Stadlan EM. Clinical diagnosis of Alzheimer's disease: report of the NINCDS-ADRDA Work Group under the auspices of Department of Health and Human Services Task Force on Alzheimer's Disease. *Neurology.* 1984;34(7):939-944.

9.	Jost BC, Grossberg GT. The evolution of psychiatric symptoms in Alzheimer's disease: a natural history study. *J Am Geriatr Soc.* 1996;44(9):1078-1081.

10.	Reitz C, Brayne C, Mayeux R. Epidemiology of Alzheimer disease. *Nat Rev Neurol.* 2011;7(3):137-152.

11.	Jack CR, Jr., Knopman DS, Jagust WJ, et al. Hypothetical model of dynamic biomarkers of the Alzheimer's pathological cascade. *Lancet Neurol.* 2010;9(1):119-128.

12.	Geldmacher DS, Whitehouse PJ. Evaluation of dementia. *N Engl J Med.* 1996;335(5):330-336.

13	Bowler JV. Vascular cognitive impairment. *J Neurol Neurosurg Psychiatry.* 1996;76:35-44.

14.	Kirshner HS. Vascular dementia: a review of recent evidence for prevention and treatment. *Curr Neurol Neurosci Rep.* 2009;9(6):437-442.

15.	Snowdon DA, Greiner LH, Mortimer JA, Riley KP, Greiner PA, Markesbery WR. Brain infarction and the clinical expression of Alzheimer disease. The Nun Study. *JAMA.* 1997;277(10):813-817.

16.	McKeith IG, Dickson DW, Lowe J, et al. Diagnosis and management of dementia with Lewy bodies: third report of the DLB Consortium. *Neurology.* 2005;65(12):1863-1872.

17.	Dodel R, Csoti I, Ebersbach G, et al. Lewy body dementia and Parkinson's disease with dementia. *J Neurol.* 2008;255 Suppl 5:39-47.

18.	Evans DA, Scherr PA, Smith LA, Albert MS, Funkenstein HH. The east Boston Alzheimer's Disease Registry. *Aging (Milano).* 1990;2(3):298-302.

19.	Alzheimer's Association. 2010 Alzheimer's disease facts and figures. *Alzheimers Dement.* 2010;6(2):158-194.

20.	Bynum JP, Rabins PV, Weller W, Niefeld M, Anderson GF, Wu AW. The relationship between a dementia diagnosis, chronic illness, Medicare expenditures, and hospital use. *J Am Geriatr Soc.* 2004;52(2):187-194.

21.	McCarthy M, Addington-Hall J, Altmann D. The experience of dying with dementia: a retrospective study. *Int J Geriatr Psychiatry.* Mar 1997;12(3):404-409.

22.	Wolfson C, Wolfson DB, Asgharian M, et al. A reevaluation of the duration of survival after the onset of dementia. *N Engl J Med.* 2001;344(15):1111-1116.

23.	Walsh JS, Welch HG, Larson EB. Survival of outpatients with Alzheimer-type dementia. *Ann Intern Med.* 1990;113(6):429-434.

24.	Rait G, Walters K, Bottomley C, Petersen I, Iliffe S, Nazareth I. Survival of people with clinical diagnosis of dementia in primary care: cohort study. *BMJ.* 2010;341:c3584.

25.	Lunney JR, Lynn J, Foley DJ, Lipson S, Guralnik JM. Patterns of functional decline at the end of life. *JAMA.* 2003;289(18):2387-2392.

26. Helmes E, Merskey H, Fox H, Fry RN, Bowler JV, Hachinski VC. Patterns of deterioration in senile dementia of the Alzheimer type. *Arch Neurol.* 1995;52(3):306-310.

27. Sands LP, Yaffe K, Lui LY, Stewart A, Eng C, Covinsky K. The effects of acute illness on ADL decline over 1 year in frail older adults with and without cognitive impairment. *J Gerontol A Biol Sci Med Sci.* 2002;57(7):M449-454.

28. Sands LP, Yaffe K, Covinsky K, et al. Cognitive screening predicts magnitude of functional recovery from admission to 3 months after discharge in hospitalized elders. *J Gerontol A Biol Sci Med Sci.* 2003;58(1):37-45.

29. Kammoun S, Gold G, Bouras C, et al. Immediate causes of death of demented and non-demented elderly. *Acta Neurol Scand Suppl.* 2000;176:96-99.

30. Burns A, Jacoby R, Luthert P, Levy R. Cause of death in Alzheimer's disease. *Age Ageing.* 1990;19(5):341-344.

31. Mitchell SL, Teno JM, Kiely DK, et al. The clinical course of advanced dementia. *N Engl J Med.* 2009;361(16):1529-1538.

32. Morrison RS, Siu AL. Survival in end-stage dementia following acute illness. *JAMA.* 2000;284(1):47-52.

33. Hanyu H, Sato T, Hirao K, Kanetaka H, Sakurai H, Iwamoto T. Differences in clinical course between dementia with Lewy bodies and Alzheimer's disease. *Eur J Neurol.* 2009;16(2):212-217.

34. Hurley AC, Volicer L. Alzheimer Disease: "It's okay, Mama, if you want to go, it's okay." *JAMA.* 2002;288(18):2324-2331.

35. Brauner DJ, Muir JC, Sachs GA. Treating nondementia illnesses in patients with dementia. *JAMA.* 2000;283(24):3230-3235.

36. Shinotoh H, Fukushi K, Nagatsuka S, et al. The amygdala and Alzheimer's disease: positron emission tomographic study of the cholinergic system. *Ann NY Acad Sci.* 2003;985:411-419.

37. Tariot PN, Federoff HJ. Current treatment for Alzheimer disease and future prospects. *Alzheimer Dis Assoc Disord.* 2003;17(Suppl 4):S105-113.

38. Winblad B, Engedal K, Soininen H, et al. A 1-year, randomized, placebo-controlled study of donepezil in patients with mild to moderate AD. *Neurology.* 2001;57(3):489-495.

39. Farlow M, Anand R, Messina J, Jr., Hartman R, Veach J. A 52-week study of the efficacy of rivastigmine in patients with mild to moderately severe Alzheimer's disease. *Eur Neurol.* 2000;44(4):236-241.

40. Raskind MA, Peskind ER, Wessel T, Yuan W. Galantamine in AD: A 6-month randomized, placebo-controlled trial with a 6-month extension. The Galantamine USA-1 Study Group. *Neurology.* 2000;54(12):2261-2268.

41. Mohs RC, Doody RS, Morris JC, et al. A 1-year, placebo-controlled preservation of function survival study of donepezil in AD patients. *Neurology.* 2001;57(3):481-488.

42. Trinh NH, Hoblyn J, Mohanty S, Yaffe K. Efficacy of cholinesterase inhibitors in the treatment of neuropsychiatric symptoms and functional impairment in Alzheimer disease: a meta-analysis. *JAMA.* 2003;289(2):210-216.

43. Katz IR, Jeste DV, Mintzer JE, Clyde C, Napolitano J, Brecher M. Comparison of risperidone and placebo for psychosis and behavioral disturbances associated with dementia: a randomized, double-blind trial. Risperidone Study Group. *J Clin Psychiatry.* 1999;60(2):107-115.

44. Howard RJ, Juszczak E, Ballard CG, et al. Donepezil for the treatment of agitation in Alzheimer's disease. *N Engl J Med.* 2007;357(14):1382-1392.

45. Becker M, Andel R, Rohrer L, Banks SM. The effect of cholinesterase inhibitors on risk of nursing home placement among medicaid beneficiaries with dementia. *Alzheimer Dis Assoc Disord.* 2006;20(3):147-152.

46. Geldmacher DS, Provenzano G, McRae T, Mastey V, Ieni JR. Donepezil is associated with delayed nursing home placement in patients with Alzheimer's disease. *J Am Geriatr Soc.* 2003;51(7):937-944.

47. Winblad B, Kilander L, Eriksson S, et al. Donepezil in patients with severe Alzheimer's disease: double-blind, parallel-group, placebo-controlled study. *Lancet.* 2006;367(9516):1057-1065.

48. Feldman H, Gauthier S, Hecker J, Vellas B, Subbiah P, Whalen E. A 24-week, randomized, double-blind study of donepezil in moderate to severe Alzheimer's disease. *Neurology.* 2001;57(4):613-620.

49. Farlow MR, Salloway S, Tariot PN, et al. Effectiveness and tolerability of high-dose (23 mg/d) versus standard-dose (10 mg/d) donepezil in moderate to severe Alzheimer's disease: a 24-week, randomized, double-blind study. *Clin Ther.* 2010;32(7):1234-1251.

50. Shega JW, Ellner L, Lau DT, Maxwell TL. Cholinesterase inhibitor and N-methyl-D-aspartic acid receptor antagonist use in older adults with end-stage dementia: a survey of hospice medical directors. *J Palliat Med*. 2009;12(9):779-783.

51. Raina P, Santaguida P, Ismaila A, et al. Effectiveness of cholinesterase inhibitors and memantine for treating dementia: evidence review for a clinical practice guideline. *Ann Intern Med*. 2008;148(5):379-397.

52. McKeith I, Del Ser T, Spano P, et al. Efficacy of rivastigmine in dementia with Lewy bodies: a randomised, double-blind, placebo-controlled international study. *Lancet*. 2000;356(9247):2031-2036.

53. Roman GC, Wilkinson DG, Doody RS, Black SE, Salloway SP, Schindler RJ. Donepezil in vascular dementia: combined analysis of two large-scale clinical trials. *Dement Geriatr Cogn Disord*. 2005;20(6):338-344.

54. Emre M, Aarsland D, Albanese A, et al. Rivastigmine for dementia associated with Parkinson's disease. *N Engl J Med*. 2004;351(24):2509-2518.

55. Courtney C, Farrell D, Gray R, et al. Long-term donepezil treatment in 565 patients with Alzheimer's disease (AD2000): randomised double-blind trial. *Lancet*. 2004;363(9427):2105-2115.

56. Danysz W, Parsons CG, Mobius HJ, Stoffler A, Quack G. Neuroprotective and symptomatological action of memantine relevant for Alzheimer's disease—a unified glutamatergic hypothesis on the mechanism of action. *Neurotox Res*. 2000;2(2-3):85-97.

57. Rogawski MA, Wenk GL. The neuropharmacological basis for the use of memantine in the treatment of Alzheimer's disease. *CNS Drug Rev*. 2003;9(3):275-308.

58. Reisberg B, Doody R, Stoffler A, Schmitt F, Ferris S, Mobius HJ. Memantine in moderate-to-severe Alzheimer's disease. *N Engl J Med*. 2003;348(14):1333-1341.

59. Tariot PN, Farlow MR, Grossberg GT, Graham SM, McDonald S, Gergel I. Memantine treatment in patients with moderate to severe Alzheimer disease already receiving donepezil: a randomized controlled trial. *JAMA*. 2004;291(3):317-324.

60. Emre M, Tsolaki M, Bonuccelli U, et al. Memantine for patients with Parkinson's disease dementia or dementia with Lewy bodies: a randomised, double-blind, placebo-controlled trial. *Lancet Neurol*. 2010;9(10):969-977.

61. Buschert V, Bokde AL, Hampel H. Cognitive intervention in Alzheimer disease. *Nat Rev Neurol*. 2010;6(9):508-517.

62. Davis RN, Massman PJ, Doody RS. Cognitive intervention in Alzheimer disease: a randomized placebo-controlled study. *Alzheimer Dis Assoc Disord*. 2001;15(1):1-9.

63. Bassuk SS, Glass TA, Berkman LF. Social disengagement and incident cognitive decline in community-dwelling elderly persons. *Ann Intern Med*. 1999;131(3):165-173.

64. Koh K, Ray R, Lee J, Nair A, Ho T, Ang PC. Dementia in elderly patients: can the 3R mental stimulation programme improve mental status? *Age Ageing*. 1994;23(3):195-199.

65. Teri L, Gibbons LE, McCurry SM, et al. Exercise plus behavioral management in patients with Alzheimer disease: a randomized controlled trial. *JAMA*. 2003;290(15):2015-2022.

66. Potter R, Ellard D, Rees K, Thorogood M. A systematic review of the effects of physical activity on physical functioning, quality of life and depression in older people with dementia. *Int J Geriatr Psychiatry*. Jan 6 2011.

67. Diesfeldt HF, van Houte LR, Moerkens RM. Duration of survival in senile dementia. *Acta Psychiatr Scand*. 1986;73(4):366-371.

68. Hanrahan P, Luchins DJ. Access to hospice programs in end-stage dementia: a national survey of hospice programs. *J Am Geriatr Soc*. 1995;43(1):56-59.

69. Doberman DJ, Yasar S, Durso SC. Would you refer this patient to hospice? An evaluation of tools for determining life expectancy in end-stage dementia. *J Palliat Med*. 2007;10(6):1410-1419.

70. Christakis NA, Escarce JJ. Survival of Medicare patients after enrollment in hospice programs. *N Engl J Med*. 1996;335(3):172-178.

71. Schonwetter RS, Han B, Small BJ, Martin B, Tope K, Haley WE. Predictors of six-month survival among patients with dementia: an evaluation of hospice Medicare guidelines. *Am J Hosp Palliat Care*. 2003;20(2):105-113.

72. Hanrahan P, Raymond M, McGowan E, Luchins DJ. Criteria for enrolling dementia patients in hospice: a replication. *Am J Hosp Palliat Care*. 1999;16(1):395-400.

73. Mitchell SL, Kiely DK, Hamel MB, Park PS, Morris JN, Fries BE. Estimating prognosis for nursing home residents with advanced dementia. *JAMA*. 2004;291(22):2734-2740.

74. Stuart B. The NHO Medical Guidelines for Non-Cancer Disease and local medical review policy: hospice access for patients with diseases other than cancer. *Hosp J*. 1999;14(3-4):139-154.

75. Mitchell SL, Miller SC, Teno JM, Kiely DK, Davis RB, Shaffer ML. Prediction of 6-month survival of nursing home residents with advanced dementia using ADEPT vs hospice eligibility guidelines. *JAMA*. 2010;304(17):1929-1935.

76. Sachs GA, Shega JW, Cox-Hayley D. Barriers to excellent end-of-life care for patients with dementia. *J Gen Intern Med*. 2004;19(10):1057-1063.

77. National Hospice and Palliative Care Organization. *NHPCO's Medical Guidelines for Determining Prognosis in Selected Non-Cancer Diseases*. 2nd ed. Arlington, VA: NHPCO; 1997.

78. Scherder E, Oosterman J, Swaab D, et al. Recent developments in pain in dementia. *BMJ*. 2005;330(7489):461-464.

79. AGS Panel on Persistent Pain in Older Persons. The management of persistent pain in older persons. *J Am Geriatr Soc*. 2002;50(6 Suppl):S205-224.

80. Taylor LJ, Herr K. Pain intensity assessment: a comparison of selected pain intensity scales for use in cognitively intact and cognitively impaired African American older adults. *Pain Manag Nurs*. 2003;4(2):87-95.

81. Shega JW, Hougham GW, Stocking CB, Cox-Hayley D, Sachs GA. Pain in community-dwelling persons with dementia: frequency, intensity, and congruence between patient and caregiver report. *J Pain Symptom Manage*. 2004;28(6):585-592.

82. Krulewitch H, London MR, Skakel VJ, Lundstedt GJ, Thomason H, Brummel-Smith K. Assessment of pain in cognitively impaired older adults: a comparison of pain assessment tools and their use by nonprofessional caregivers. *J Am Geriatr Soc*. 2000;48(12):1607-1611.

83. Ferrell BA. Pain evaluation and management in the nursing home. *Ann Intern Med*. 1995;123(9):681-687.

84. Won A, Lapane K, Gambassi G, Bernabei R, Mor V, Lipsitz LA. Correlates and management of nonmalignant pain in the nursing home. SAGE Study Group. Systematic Assessment of Geriatric drug use via Epidemiology. *J Am Geriatr Soc*. 1999;47(8):936-942.

85. Hootman J, Bolen J, Helmick C, Langmaid G. Prevalence of doctor-diagnosed arthritis. Available at: www.cdc.gov/mmwr/preview/mmwrhtml/mm5540a2.htm. Accessed December 28, 2006.

86. Keenan AM, Tennant A, Fear J, Emery P, Conaghan PG. Impact of multiple joint problems on daily living tasks in people in the community over age fifty-five. *Arthritis Rheum*. 2006;55(5):757-764.

87. Parmelee PA. Pain in cognitively impaired older persons. *Clin Geriatr Med*. 1996;12(3):473-487.

88. Hurley AC, Volicer BJ, Hanrahan PA, Houde S, Volicer L. Assessment of discomfort in advanced Alzheimer patients. *Res Nurs Health*. 1992;15(5):369-377.

89. Herr K, Bursch H, Ersek M, Miller LL, Swafford K. Use of pain-behavioral assessment tools in the nursing home: expert consensus recommendations for practice. *J Gerontol Nurs*. 2010;36(3):18-29.

90. Feldt KS. The checklist of nonverbal pain indicators (CNPI). *Pain Manag Nurs*. 2000;1(1):13-21.

91. Shega JW, Rudy T, Keefe FJ, Perri LC, Mengin OT, Weiner DK. Validity of pain behaviors in persons with mild to moderate cognitive impairment. *J Am Geriatr Soc*. 2008;56(9):1631-1637.

92. Elliott AF, Horgas AL. Effects of an analgesic trial in reducing pain behaviors in community-dwelling older adults with dementia. *Nurs Res*. 2009;58(2):140-145.

93. Manfredi PL, Breuer B, Wallenstein S, Stegmann M, Bottomley G, Libow L. Opioid treatment for agitation in patients with advanced dementia. *Int J Geriatr Psychiatry*. 2003;18(8):700-705.

94. Ersek M, Cherrier MM, Overman SS, Irving GA. The cognitive effects of opioids. *Pain Manag Nurs*. 2004;5(2):75-93.

95. Morrison RS, Magaziner J, Gilbert M, et al. Relationship between pain and opioid analgesics on the development of delirium following hip fracture. *J Gerontol A Biol Sci Med Sci*. 2003;58(1):76-81.

96. Hollingworth P, Hamshere ML, Moskvina V, et al. Four components describe behavioral symptoms in 1,120 individuals with late-onset Alzheimer's disease. *J Am Geriatr Soc*. 2006;54(9):1348-1354.

97. Spalletta G, Musicco M, Padovani A, et al. Neuropsychiatric symptoms and syndromes in a large cohort of newly diagnosed, untreated patients with Alzheimer disease. *Am J Geriatr Psychiatry*. 2010;18(11):1026-1035.

98. Murman DL, Colenda CC. The economic impact of neuropsychiatric symptoms in Alzheimer's disease: can drugs ease the burden? *Pharmacoeconomics*. 2005;23(3):227-242.

99. McGivney SA, Mulvihill M, Taylor B. Validating the GDS depression screen in the nursing home. *J Am Geriatr Soc*. 1994;42(5):490-492.

100. Gerety MB, Williams JW, Jr., Mulrow CD, et al. Performance of case-finding tools for depression in the nursing home: influence of clinical and functional characteristics and selection of optimal threshold scores. *J Am Geriatr Soc*. 1994;42(10):1103-1109.

101. Alexopoulos GS, Abrams RC, Young RC, Shamoian CA. Cornell Scale for Depression in Dementia. *Biol Psychiatry*. 1988;23(3):271-284.

102. Ballard CG, Patel A, Solis M, Lowe K, Wilcock G. A one-year follow-up study of depression in dementia sufferers. *Br J Psychiatry*. 1996;168(3):287-291.

103. Gruber-Baldini AL, Zimmerman S, Boustani M, Watson LC, Williams CS, Reed PS. Characteristics associated with depression in long-term care residents with dementia. *Gerontologist*. 2005;45(1):50-55.

104. Zubenko GS, Zubenko WN, McPherson S, et al. A collaborative study of the emergence and clinical features of the major depressive syndrome of Alzheimer's disease. *Am J Psychiatry*. 2003;160(5):857-866.

105. Karttunen K, Karppi P, Hiltunen A, et al. Neuropsychiatric symptoms and quality of life in patients with very mild and mild Alzheimer's disease. *Int J Geriatr Psychiatry*. 2011;26(5):473-482.

106. Forstl H, Burns A, Luthert P, Cairns N, Lantos P, Levy R. Clinical and neuropathological correlates of depression in Alzheimer's disease. *Psychol Med*. 1992;22(4):877-884.

107. Bains J, Birks JS, Dening TR. The efficacy of antidepressants in the treatment of depression in dementia. *Cochrane Database Syst Rev*. 2002;(4):CD003944.

108. Modrego PJ. Depression in Alzheimer's disease. Pathophysiology, diagnosis, and treatment. *J Alzheimers Dis*. 2010;21(4):1077-1087.

109. Katz IR, Simpson GM, Curlik SM, Parmelee PA, Muhly C. Pharmacologic treatment of major depression for elderly patients in residential care settings. *J Clin Psychiatry*. 1990;51 Suppl:41-47, discussion 48.

110. Galynker I, Ieronimo C, Miner C, Rosenblum J, Vilkas N, Rosenthal R. Methylphenidate treatment of negative symptoms in patients with dementia. *J Neuropsychiatry Clin Neurosci*. 1997;9(2):231-239.

111. Dolder CR, Davis LN, McKinsey J. Use of psychostimulants in patients with dementia. *Ann Pharmacother*. 2010;44(10):1624-1632.

112. Snowden M, Sato K, Roy-Byrne P. Assessment and treatment of nursing home residents with depression or behavioral symptoms associated with dementia: a review of the literature. *J Am Geriatr Soc*. 2003;51(9):1305-1317.

113. Hausner L, Damian M, Sartorius A, Frolich L. Efficacy and cognitive side effects of electroconvulsive therapy (ECT) in depressed elderly inpatients with coexisting mild cognitive impairment or dementia. *J Clin Psychiatry*. 2011;72(1):91-97.

114. Landes AM, Sperry SD, Strauss ME. Prevalence of apathy, dysphoria, and depression in relation to dementia severity in Alzheimer's disease. *J Neuropsychiatry Clin Neurosci*. 2005;17(3):342-349.

115. Landes AM, Sperry SD, Strauss ME, Geldmacher DS. Apathy in Alzheimer's disease. *J Am Geriatr Soc*. 2001;49(12):1700-1707.

116. Holmes C, Wilkinson D, Dean C, et al. The efficacy of donepezil in the treatment of neuropsychiatric symptoms in Alzheimer disease. *Neurology*. 2004;63(2):214-219.

117. Peters KR, Rockwood K, Black SE, et al. Characterizing neuropsychiatric symptoms in subjects referred to dementia clinics. *Neurology*. 2006;66(4):523-528.

118. Craig D, Mirakhur A, Hart DJ, McIlroy SP, Passmore AP. A cross-sectional study of neuropsychiatric symptoms in 435 patients with Alzheimer's disease. *Am J Geriatr Psychiatry*. 2005;13(6):460-468.

119. Lyketsos CG, Lopez O, Jones B, Fitzpatrick AL, Breitner J, DeKosky S. Prevalence of neuropsychiatric symptoms in dementia and mild cognitive impairment: results from the cardiovascular health study. *JAMA*. 2002;288(12):1475-1483.

120. Del Ser T, McKeith I, Anand R, Cicin-Sain A, Ferrara R, Spiegel R. Dementia with lewy bodies: findings from an international multicentre study. *Int J Geriatr Psychiatry*. 2000;15(11):1034-1045.

121. Ropacki SA, Jeste DV. Epidemiology of and risk factors for psychosis of Alzheimer's disease: a review of 55 studies published from 1990 to 2003. *Am J Psychiatry*. 2005;162(11):2022-2030.

122. Paulsen JS, Salmon DP, Thal LJ, et al. Incidence of and risk factors for hallucinations and delusions in patients with probable AD. *Neurology.* 2000;54(10):1965-1971.

123. Schneider LS, Tariot PN, Dagerman KS, et al. Effectiveness of atypical antipsychotic drugs in patients with Alzheimer's disease. *N Engl J Med.* 2006;355(15):1525-1538.

124. Carson S, McDonagh MS, Peterson K. A systematic review of the efficacy and safety of atypical antipsychotics in patients with psychological and behavioral symptoms of dementia. *J Am Geriatr Soc.* 2006;54(2):354-361.

125. Schneider LS, Dagerman K, Insel PS. Efficacy and adverse effects of atypical antipsychotics for dementia: meta-analysis of randomized, placebo-controlled trials. *Am J Geriatr Psychiatry.* 2006;14(3):191-210.

126. Rosenheck RA, Leslie DL, Sindelar JL, et al. Cost-benefit analysis of second-generation antipsychotics and placebo in a randomized trial of the treatment of psychosis and aggression in Alzheimer disease. *Arch Gen Psychiatry.* 2007;64(11):1259-1268.

127. Jeste DV, Blazer D, Casey D, et al. ACNP White Paper: update on use of antipsychotic drugs in elderly persons with dementia. *Neuropsychopharmacology.* 2008;33(5):957-970.

128. Schneider LS, Dagerman KS, Insel P. Risk of death with atypical antipsychotic drug treatment for dementia: meta-analysis of randomized placebo-controlled trials. *JAMA.* 2005;294(15):1934-1943.

129. Ballard CG, Gauthier S, Cummings JL, et al. Management of agitation and aggression associated with Alzheimer disease. *Nat Rev Neurol.* 2009;5(5):245-255.

130. Jeste DV, Meeks TW, Kim DS, Zubenko GS. Research agenda for DSM-V: diagnostic categories and criteria for neuropsychiatric syndromes in dementia. *J Geriatr Psychiatry Neurol.* 2006;19(3):160-171.

131. Hooker K, Bowman SR, Coehlo DP, et al. Behavioral change in persons with dementia: relationships with mental and physical health of caregivers. *J Gerontol B Psychol Sci Soc Sci.* 2002;57(5):P453-460.

132. Cohen-Mansfield J, Marx MS, Werner P. Agitation in elderly persons: an integrative report of findings in a nursing home. *Int Psychogeriatr.* 1992;4 Suppl 2:221-240.

133. Hope T, Keene J, Fairburn C, McShane R, Jacoby R. Behaviour changes in dementia: are there behavioural syndromes? *Int J Geriatr Psychiatry.* 1997;12(11):1074-1078.

134. Hamel M, Gold DP, Andres D, et al. Predictors and consequences of aggressive behavior by community-based dementia patients. *Gerontologist.* 1990;30(2):206-211.

135. Deutsch LH, Bylsma FW, Rovner BW, Steele C, Folstein MF. Psychosis and physical aggression in probable Alzheimer's disease. *Am J Psychiatry.* 1991;148(9):1159-1163.

136. McMinn B, Draper B. Vocally disruptive behaviour in dementia: development of an evidence based practice guideline. *Aging Ment Health.* 2005;9(1):16-24.

137. Ayalon L, Gum AM, Feliciano L, Arean PA. Effectiveness of nonpharmacological interventions for the management of neuropsychiatric symptoms in patients with dementia: a systematic review. *Arch Intern Med.* 2006;166(20):2182-2188.

138. Gitlin LN, Winter L, Dennis MP, Hodgson N, Hauck WW. Targeting and managing behavioral symptoms in individuals with dementia: a randomized trial of a nonpharmacological intervention. *J Am Geriatr Soc.* 2010;58(8):1465-1474.

139. Cohen-Mansfield J, Marx MS, Dakheel-Ali M, Regier NG, Thein K, Freedman L. Can agitated behavior of nursing home residents with dementia be prevented with the use of standardized stimuli? *J Am Geriatr Soc.* 2010;58(8):1459-1464.

140. Martinon-Torres G, Fioravanti M, Grimley EJ. Trazodone for agitation in dementia. *Cochrane Database Syst Rev.* 2004(4):CD004990.

141. Sultzer DL, Gray KF, Gunay I, Berisford MA, Mahler ME. A double-blind comparison of trazodone and haloperidol for treatment of agitation in patients with dementia. *Am J Geriatr Psychiatry.* 1997;5(1):60-69.

142. Pollock BG, Mulsant BH, Rosen J, et al. Comparison of citalopram, perphenazine, and placebo for the acute treatment of psychosis and behavioral disturbances in hospitalized, demented patients. *Am J Psychiatry.* 2002;159(3):460-465.

143. Gauthier S, Wirth Y, Mobius HJ. Effects of memantine on behavioural symptoms in Alzheimer's disease patients: an analysis of the Neuropsychiatric Inventory (NPI) data of two randomised, controlled studies. *Int J Geriatr Psychiatry.* 2005;20(5):459-464.

144. Kirven LE, Montero EF. Comparison of thioridazine and diazepam in the control of nonpsychotic symptoms associated with senility: double-blind study. *J Am Geriatr Soc.* 1973;21(12):546-551.

145. Lonergan ET, Cameron M, Luxenberg J. Valproic acid for agitation in dementia. *Cochrane Database Syst Rev.* 2004(2):CD003945.

146. Tariot PN, Erb R, Podgorski CA, et al. Efficacy and tolerability of carbamazepine for agitation and aggression in dementia. *Am J Psychiatry.* 1998;155(1):54-61.

147. Miller LJ. Gabapentin for treatment of behavioral and psychological symptoms of dementia. *Ann Pharmacother.* 2001;35(4):427-431.

148. Ganguli M, Rodriguez EG. Reporting of dementia on death certificates: a community study. *J Am Geriatr Soc.* 1999;47(7):842-849.

149. Mitchell SL, Kiely DK, Hamel MB. Dying with advanced dementia in the nursing home. *Arch Intern Med.* 2004;164(3):321-326.

150. Mitchell SL, Morris JN, Park PS, Fries BE. Terminal care for persons with advanced dementia in the nursing home and home care settings. *J Palliat Med.* 2004;7(6):808-816.

151. Baer WM, Hanson LC. Families' perception of the added value of hospice in the nursing home. *J Am Geriatr Soc.* 2000;48(8):879-882.

152. Munn JC, Hanson LC, Zimmerman S, Sloane PD, Mitchell CM. Is hospice associated with improved end-of-life care in nursing homes and assisted living facilities? *J Am Geriatr Soc.* 2006;54(3):490-495.

153. Miller SC, Mor V, Teno J. Hospice enrollment and pain assessment and management in nursing homes. *J Pain Symptom Manage.* 2003;26(3):791-799.

154. Shega JW, Hougham GW, Stocking CB, Cox-Hayley D, Sachs GA. Management of noncancer pain in community-dwelling persons with dementia. *J Am Geriatr Soc.* 2006;54(12):1892-1897.

155. Volicer L, Seltzer B, Rheaume Y, et al. Eating difficulties in patients with probable dementia of the Alzheimer type. *J Geriatr Psychiatry Neurol.* 1989;2(4):188-195.

156. Volicer L, Rheaume Y, Cyr D. Treatment of depression in advanced Alzheimer's disease using sertraline. *J Geriatr Psychiatry Neurol.* 1994;7(4):227-229.

157. Bosley BN, Weiner DK, Rudy TE, Granieri E. Is chronic nonmalignant pain associated with decreased appetite in older adults? Preliminary evidence. *J Am Geriatr Soc.* 2004;52(2):247-251.

158. Callahan CM, Haag KM, Weinberger M, et al. Outcomes of percutaneous endoscopic gastrostomy among older adults in a community setting. *J Am Geriatr Soc.* 2000;48(9):1048-1054.

159. Finucane TE, Christmas C, Travis K. Tube feeding in patients with advanced dementia: a review of the evidence. *JAMA.* 1999;282(14):1365-1370.

160. Gillick MR. Rethinking the role of tube feeding in patients with advanced dementia. *N Engl J Med.* 2000;342(3):206-210.

161. Shega JW, Hougham GW, Stocking CB, Cox-Hayley D, Sachs GA. Barriers to limiting the practice of feeding tube placement in advanced dementia. *J Palliat Med.* 2003;6(6):885-893.

162. Candy B, Sampson EL, Jones L. Enteral tube feeding in older people with advanced dementia: findings from a Cochrane systematic review. *Int J Palliat Nurs.* 2009;15(8):396-404.

163. Meier DE, Ahronheim JC, Morris J, Baskin-Lyons S, Morrison RS. High short-term mortality in hospitalized patients with advanced dementia: lack of benefit of tube feeding. *Arch Intern Med.* 2001;161(4):594-599.

164. Kuo S, Rhodes RL, Mitchell SL, Mor V, Teno JM. Natural history of feeding-tube use in nursing home residents with advanced dementia. *J Am Med Dir Assoc.* 2009;10(4):264-270.

165. Finucane TE, Bynum JP. Use of tube feeding to prevent aspiration pneumonia. *Lancet.* 1996;348(9039):1421-1424.

166. Volandes AE, Paasche-Orlow MK, Barry MJ, et al. Video decision support tool for advance care planning in dementia: randomised controlled trial. *BMJ.* 2009;338:b2159.

167. Morrison RS, Ahronheim JC, Morrison GR, et al. Pain and discomfort associated with common hospital procedures and experiences. *J Pain Symptom Manage.* 1998;15(2):91-101.

168. van der Steen JT, Kruse RL, Ooms ME, et al. Treatment of nursing home residents with dementia and lower respiratory tract infection in the United States and The Netherlands: an ocean apart. *J Am Geriatr Soc.* 2004;52(5):691-699.

169. Fabiszewski KJ, Volicer B, Volicer L. Effect of antibiotic treatment on outcome of fevers in institutionalized Alzheimer patients. *JAMA* 1990;263(23):3168-31/2.

170. Givens JL, Jones RN, Shaffer ML, Kiely DK, Mitchell SL. Survival and comfort after treatment of pneumonia in advanced dementia. *Arch Intern Med.* 2010;170(13):1102-1107.

171. Morrison RS, Siu AL. A comparison of pain and its treatment in advanced dementia and cognitively intact patients with hip fracture. *J Pain Symptom Manage.* 2000;19(4):240-248.

172. Feldt KS, Ryden MB, Miles S. Treatment of pain in cognitively impaired compared with cognitively intact older patients with hip-fracture. *J Am Geriatr Soc.* 1998;46(9):1079-1085.

173. Alexander GC, Sayla MA, Holmes HM, Sachs GA. Prioritizing and stopping prescription medicines. *CMAJ.* 2006;174(8):1083-1084.

174. Holmes HM, Hayley DC, Alexander GC, Sachs GA. Reconsidering medication appropriateness for patients late in life. *Arch Intern Med.* 2006;166(6):605-609.

175. Volicer L, Rheaume Y, Brown J, Fabiszewski K, Brady R. Hospice approach to the treatment of patients with advanced dementia of the Alzheimer type. *JAMA.* 1986;256(16):2210-2213.

176. Shega JW, Hougham GW, Stocking CB, Cox-Hayley D, Sachs GA. Patients dying with dementia: experience at the end of life and impact of hospice care. *J Pain Symptom Manage.* 2008;35(5):499-507.

177. Schulz R, Mendelsohn AB, Haley WE, et al. End-of-life care and the effects of bereavement on family caregivers of persons with dementia. *N Engl J Med.* 2003;349(20):1936-1942.

178. Miller SC, Mor V, Wu N, Gozalo P, Lapane K. Does receipt of hospice care in nursing homes improve the management of pain at the end of life? *J Am Geriatr Soc.* 2002;50(3):507-515.

179. Kiely DK, Givens JL, Shaffer ML, Teno JM, Mitchell SL. Hospice use and outcomes in nursing home residents with advanced dementia. *J Am Geriatr Soc.* 2010;58(12):2284-2291.

180. Ory MG, Hoffman RR, 3rd, Yee JL, Tennstedt S, Schulz R. Prevalence and impact of caregiving: a detailed comparison between dementia and nondementia caregivers. *Gerontologist.* 1999;39(2):177-185.

181. Schulz R, Newsom J, Mittelmark M, Burton L, Hirsch C, Jackson S. Health effects of caregiving: the caregiver health effects study: an ancillary study of the Cardiovascular Health Study. *Ann Behav Med.* 1997;19(2):110-116.

182. Mahoney R, Regan C, Katona C, Livingston G. Anxiety and depression in family caregivers of people with Alzheimer disease: the LASER-AD study. *Am J Geriatr Psychiatry.* 2005;13(9):795-801.

183. Schulz R, Beach SR. Caregiving as a risk factor for mortality: the Caregiver Health Effects Study. *JAMA.* 1999;282(23):2215-2219.

184. Yee JL, Schulz R. Gender differences in psychiatric morbidity among family caregivers: a review and analysis. *Gerontologist.* 2000;40(2):147-164.

185. Yaffe K, Fox P, Newcomer R, et al. Patient and caregiver characteristics and nursing home placement in patients with dementia. *JAMA.* 2002;287(16):2090-2097.

186. Schulz R, Belle SH, Czaja SJ, McGinnis KA, Stevens A, Zhang S. Long-term care placement of dementia patients and caregiver health and well-being. *JAMA.* 2004;292(8):961-967.

187. Gitlin LN, Belle SH, Burgio LD, et al. Effect of multicomponent interventions on caregiver burden and depression: the REACH multisite initiative at 6-month follow-up. *Psychol Aging.* 2003;18(3):361-374.

188. Rabinowitz YG, Mausbach BT, Coon DW, Depp C, Thompson LW, Gallagher-Thompson D. The moderating effect of self-efficacy on intervention response in women family caregivers of older adults with dementia. *Am J Geriatr Psychiatry.* 2006;14(8):642-649.

189. Belle SH, Burgio L, Burns R, et al. Enhancing the quality of life of dementia caregivers from different ethnic or racial groups: a randomized, controlled trial. *Ann Intern Med.* 2006;145(10):727-738.

190. Elliott AF, Burgio LD, Decoster J. Enhancing caregiver health: findings from the resources for enhancing Alzheimer's caregiver health II intervention. *J Am Geriatr Soc.* 2010;58(1):30-37.

191. Sorensen S, Pinquart M, Duberstein P. How effective are interventions with caregivers? An updated meta-analysis. *Gerontologist.* 2002;42(3):356-372.

192. Schulz R, Boerner K, Shear K, Zhang S, Gitlin LN. Predictors of complicated grief among dementia caregivers: a prospective study of bereavement. *Am J Geriatr Psychiatry.* 2006;14(8):650-658.

193. Mannino DM, Buist AS. Global burden of COPD: risk factors, prevalence, and future trends. *Lancet.* 2007;370(9589):765-773.

194. Afonso AS, Verhamme KM, Sturkenboom MC, Brusselle GG. COPD in the general population: prevalence, incidence and survival. *Respir Med.* 2011;105(12):1872-1884.

195. Soriano JB, Rodriguez-Roisin R. Chronic obstructive pulmonary disease overview: epidemiology, risk factors, and clinical presentation. *Proceedings of the American Thoracic Society.* 2011;8(4):363-367.

196. Jemal A, Ward E, Hao Y, Thun M. Trends in the leading causes of death in the United States, 1970-2002. *JAMA.* 2005;294(10):1255-1259.

197. Centers for Disease Control and Prevention. Deaths from chronic obstructive pulmonary disease: United States, 2000-2005. Available at: www.cdc.gov/mmwr/preview/mmwrhtml/mm5745a.htm. Accessed April 7, 2011.

198. Lacasse Y, Brooks D, Goldstein RS. Trends in the epidemiology of COPD in Canada, 1980 to 1995. COPD and Rehabilitation Committee of the Canadian Thoracic Society. *Chest.* 1999;116(2):306-313.

199. Canadian Institute for Health Information, Canadian Lung Association, Health Canada, Statistics Canada. Respiratory disease in Canada. [Public Health Agency of Canada Website]. Available at: www.phac-aspc.gc.ca/publicat/rdc-mrc01/index.html. Accessed February 27, 2012.

200. Murray CJ, Lopez AD. Mortality by cause for eight regions of the world: Global Burden of Disease Study. *Lancet.* 1997;349(9061):1269-1276.

201. Raherison C, Girodet PO. Epidemiology of COPD. *Eur Respir Rev.* 2009;18(114):213-221.

202. Fletcher MJ, Upton J, Taylor-Fishwick J, et al. COPD uncovered: an international survey on the impact of chronic obstructive pulmonary disease [COPD] on a working age population. *BMC Public Health.* 2011;11:612.

203. Lynn J, Ely EW, Zhong Z, et al. Living and dying with chronic obstructive pulmonary disease. *J Am Geriatr Soc.* 2000;48(5 Suppl):S91-100.

204. Lynn J, Teno JM, Phillips RS, et al. Perceptions by family members of the dying experience of older and seriously ill patients. SUPPORT Investigators. Study to Understand Prognoses and Preferences for Outcomes and Risks of Treatments. *Ann Intern Med.* 1997;126(2):97-106.

205. Patil SP, Krishnan JA, Lechtzin N, Diette GB. In-hospital mortality following acute exacerbations of chronic obstructive pulmonary disease. *Arch Intern Med.* 2003;163(10):1180-1186.

206. Connors AF, Jr., Dawson NV, Thomas C, et al. Outcomes following acute exacerbation of severe chronic obstructive lung disease. The SUPPORT investigators (Study to Understand Prognoses and Preferences for Outcomes and Risks of Treatments). *Am J Respir Crit Care Med.* 1996;154(4 Pt 1):959-967.

207. Au DH, Udris EM, Fihn SD, McDonell MB, Curtis JR. Differences in health care utilization at the end of life among patients with chronic obstructive pulmonary disease and patients with lung cancer. *Arch Intern Med.* 2006;166(3):326-331.

208. Edmonds P, Karlsen S, Khan S, Addington-Hall J. A comparison of the palliative care needs of patients dying from chronic respiratory diseases and lung cancer. *Palliat Med.* 2001;15(4):287-295.

209. Claessens MT, Lynn J, Zhong Z, et al. Dying with lung cancer or chronic obstructive pulmonary disease: insights from SUPPORT. Study to Understand Prognoses and Preferences for Outcomes and Risks of Treatments. *J Am Geriatr Soc.* 2000;48(5 Suppl):S146-153.

210. Bailey PH. The dyspnea-anxiety-dyspnea cycle—COPD patients' stories of breathlessness: "It's scary/when you can't breathe." *Qual Health Res.* 2004;14(6):760-778.

211. Jones I, Kirby A, Ormiston P, et al. The needs of patients dying of chronic obstructive pulmonary disease in the community. *Fam Pract.* 2004;21(3):310-313.

212. Elkington H, White P, Addington-Hall J, Higgs R, Edmonds P. The healthcare needs of chronic obstructive pulmonary disease patients in the last year of life. *Palliat Med.* 2005;19(6):485-491.

213. Elkington H, White P, Addington-Hall J, Higgs R, Pettinari C. The last year of life of COPD: a qualitative study of symptoms and services. *Respir Med.* 2004;98(5):439-445.

214. Miravitlles M, Naberan K, Cantoni J, Azpeitia A. Socioeconomic status and health-related quality of life of patients with chronic obstructive pulmonary disease. *Respiration.* 2011;82(5):402-408.

215. Curtis JR, Deyo RA, Hudson LD. Pulmonary rehabilitation in chronic respiratory insufficiency. Health-related quality of life among patients with chronic obstructive pulmonary disease. *Thorax.* 1994;49(2):162-170.

216. O'Donnell DE, Banzett RB, Carrieri-Kohlman V, et al. Pathophysiology of dyspnea in chronic obstructive pulmonary disease: a roundtable. *Proc Am Thorac Soc.* 2007;4(2):145-168.

217. Nishino T. Dyspnoea: underlying mechanisms and treatment. *Br J Anaesth.* 2011;106(4):463-474.

218. Evans KC, Banzett RB, Adams L, McKay L, Frackowiak RS, Corfield DR. BOLD fMRI identifies limbic, paralimbic, and cerebellar activation during air hunger. *J Neurophysiol.* 2002;88(3):1500-1511.

219. Harper RM. Visualization of neural activity associated with dyspnea. *Am J Respir Crit Care Med.* 2001;163(4):805-806.

220. Aaron SD, Vandemheen KL, Fergusson D, et al. Tiotropium in combination with placebo, salmeterol, or fluticasone-salmeterol for treatment of chronic obstructive pulmonary disease: a randomized trial. *Ann Intern Med.* 2007;146(8):545-555.

221. Ko FW, Tam W, Tung AH, et al. A longitudinal study of serial BODE indices in predicting mortality and readmissions for COPD. *Respir Med.* 2011;105(2):266-273.

222. Marin JM, Cote CG, Diaz O, et al. Prognostic assessment in COPD: health related quality of life and the BODE index. *Respir Med.* 2011;105(6):916-921.

223. Tranmer JE, Heyland D, Dudgeon D, Groll D, Squires-Graham M, Coulson K. Measuring the symptom experience of seriously ill cancer and noncancer hospitalized patients near the end of life with the memorial symptom assessment scale. *J Pain Symptom Manage.* 2003;25(5):420-429.

224. Gore JM, Brophy CJ, Greenstone MA. How well do we care for patients with end stage chronic obstructive pulmonary disease (COPD)? A comparison of palliative care and quality of life in COPD and lung cancer. *Thorax.* 2000;55(12):1000-1006.

225. Rocker GM, Dodek PM, Heyland DK. Toward optimal end-of-life care for patients with advanced chronic obstructive pulmonary disease: insights from a multicentre study. *Can Respir J.* 2008;15(5):249-254.

226. White P, White S, Edmonds P, et al. Palliative care or end-of-life care in advanced chronic obstructive pulmonary disease; a prospective community survey. *Br J Gen Pract.* 2011;61(587):e362-370.

227. Shah S, Blanchard M, Tookman A, Jones L, Blizard R, King M. Estimating needs in life threatening illness: a feasibility study to assess the views of patients and doctors. *Palliat Med.* 2006;20(3):205-210.

228. O'Donnell DE, Aaron S, Bourbeau J, et al. Canadian Thoracic Society recommendations for management of chronic obstructive pulmonary disease--2003. *Can Respir J.* 2003;10 Suppl A:11A-65A.

229. Abrahm JL, Hansen-Flaschen J. Hospice care for patients with advanced lung disease. *Chest.* 2002;121(1):220-229.

230. Elkington H, White P, Higgs R, Pettinari CJ. GPs' views of discussions of prognosis in severe COPD. *Fam Pract.* 2001;18(4):440-444.

231. Guthrie SJ, Hill KM, Muers ME. Living with severe COPD. A qualitative exploration of the experience of patients in Leeds. *Respir Med.* 2001;95(3):196-204.

232. Selecky PA, Eliasson CA, Hall RI, Schneider RF, Varkey B, McCaffree DR. Palliative and end-of-life care for patients with cardiopulmonary diseases: American College of Chest Physicians position statement. *Chest.* 2005;128(5):3599-3610.

233. Fried TR, Bradley EH. What matters to seriously ill older persons making end-of-life treatment decisions? A qualitative study. *J Palliat Med.* 2003;6(2):237-244.

234. Oliver SM. Living with failing lungs: the doctor-patient relationship. *Fam Pract.* 2001;18(4):430-439.

235. Santo Tomas LH, Varkey B. Improving health-related quality of life in chronic obstructive pulmonary disease. *Curr Opin Pulm Med.* 2004;10(2):120-127.

236. Mulcahy P, Buetow S, Osman L, et al. GPs' attitudes to discussing prognosis in severe COPD: an Auckland (NZ) to London (UK) comparison. *Fam Pract.* 2005;22(5):538-540.

237. Knauft E, Nielsen EL, Engelberg RA, Patrick DL, Curtis JR. Barriers and facilitators to end-of-life care communication for patients with COPD. *Chest.* 2005;127(6):2188-2196.

238. Grbich C, Maddocks I, Parker D, et al. Identification of patients with noncancer diseases for palliative care services. *Palliat Support Care.* 2005;3(1):5-14.

239. Coventry PA, Grande GE, Richards DA, Todd CJ. Prediction of appropriate timing of palliative care for older adults with non-malignant life-threatening disease: a systematic review. *Age Ageing.* 2005;34(3):218-227.

240. Murray SA, Boyd K, Kendall M, Worth A, Benton TF, Clausen H. Dying of lung cancer or cardiac failure: prospective qualitative interview study of patients and their carers in the community. *BMJ.* 2002;325(7370):929.

241. Hansen-Flaschen J. Chronic obstructive pulmonary disease: the last year of life. *Respir Care.* 2004;49(1):90-97; discussion 97-98.

242. Almagro P, Calbo E, Ochoa de Echaguen A, et al. Mortality after hospitalization for COPD. *Chest.* 2002;121(5):1441-1448.

243. Domingo-Salvany A, Lamarca R, Ferrer M, et al. Health-related quality of life and mortality in male patients with chronic obstructive pulmonary disease. *Am J Respir Crit Care Med.* 2002;166(5):680-685.

244. Fan VS, Curtis JR, Tu SP, McDonell MB, Fihn SD. Using quality of life to predict hospitalization and mortality in patients with obstructive lung diseases. *Chest.* 2002;122(2):429-436.

245. Nishimura K, Izumi T, Tsukino M, Oga T. Dyspnea is a better predictor of 5-year survival than airway obstruction in patients with COPD. *Chest.* 2002;121(5):1434-1440.

246. Celli BR, Cote CG, Marin JM, et al. The body-mass index, airflow obstruction, dyspnea, and exercise capacity index in chronic obstructive pulmonary disease. *N Engl J Med.* 2004;350(10):1005-1012.

247. Martinez FJ, Foster G, Curtis JL, et al. Predictors of mortality in patients with emphysema and severe airflow obstruction. *Am J Respir Crit Care Med.* 2006;173(12):1326-1334.

248. Soler-Cataluna JJ, Martinez-Garcia MA, Roman Sanchez P, Salcedo E, Navarro M, Ochando R. Severe acute exacerbations and mortality in patients with chronic obstructive pulmonary disease. *Thorax.* 2005;60(11):925-931.

249. Criner GJ, Cordova F, Sternberg AL, Martinez FJ. The National Emphysema Treatment Trial (NETT): part I: lessons learned about emphysema. *Am J Respir Crit Care Med.* 2011;184(7):763-770.

250. Nussbaumer-Ochsner Y, Rabe KF. Systemic manifestations of COPD. *Chest.* 2011;139(1):165-173.

251. Casaburi R, ZuWallack R. Pulmonary rehabilitation for management of chronic obstructive pulmonary disease. *N Engl J Med.* 2009;360(13):1329-1335.

252. Eisner MD, Iribarren C, Blanc PD, et al. Development of disability in chronic obstructive pulmonary disease: beyond lung function. *Thorax.* 2011;66(2):108-114.

253. Terzano C, Conti V, Di Stefano F, et al. Comorbidity, hospitalization, and mortality in COPD: results from a longitudinal study. *Lung.* 2010;188(4):321-329.

254. Rocker GM, Sinuff T, Horton R, Hernandez P. Advanced chronic obstructive pulmonary disease: innovative approaches to palliation. *J Palliat Med.* 2007;10(3):783-797.

255. Han MK, Martinez FJ. Pharmacotherapeutic approaches to preventing acute exacerbations of chronic obstructive pulmonary disease. *Proceedings of the American Thoracic Society.* Aug 2011;8(4):356-362.

256. Ginsburg ME, Thomashow BM, Yip CK, et al. Lung volume reduction surgery using the NETT selection criteria. *Ann Thorac Surg.* 2011;91(5):1556-1560.

257. Jennings AL, Davies AN, Higgins JP, Gibbs JS, Broadley KE. A systematic review of the use of opioids in the management of dyspnoea. *Thorax.* 2002;57(11):939-944.

258. Marciniuk D, Goodridge D, Hernandez P, et al. Managing dyspnea in patients with advanced chronic obstructive pulmonary disease: A Canadian Thoracic Society clinical practice guideline. *Can Respir J.* 2011;18(2):69-78.

259. Calverley PM, Anderson JA, Celli B, et al. Salmeterol and fluticasone propionate and survival in chronic obstructive pulmonary disease. *N Engl J Med.* 2007;356(8):775-789.

260. Tashkin DP, Cooper CB. The role of long-acting bronchodilators in the management of stable COPD. *Chest.* 2004;125(1):249-259.

261. Tashkin DP, Celli B, Senn S, et al. A 4-year trial of tiotropium in chronic obstructive pulmonary disease. *N Engl J Med.* 2008;359(15):1543-1554.

262. Singh S, Loke YK, Furberg CD. Inhaled anticholinergics and risk of major adverse cardiovascular events in patients with chronic obstructive pulmonary disease: a systematic review and meta-analysis. *JAMA.* 2008;300(12):1439-1450.

263. Adams SG, Anzueto A, Briggs DD, Jr., Leimer I, Kesten S. Evaluation of withdrawal of maintenance tiotropium in COPD. *Respir Med.* 2009;103(10):1415-1420.

264. Qaseem A, Wilt TJ, Weinberger SE, et al. Diagnosis and management of stable chronic obstructive pulmonary disease: a clinical practice guideline update from the American College of Physicians, American College of Chest Physicians, American Thoracic Society, and European Respiratory Society. *Ann Intern Med.* 2011;155(3):179-191.

265. Nuhoglu Y, Nuhoglu C. Aminophylline for treating asthma and chronic obstructive pulmonary disease. *Expert Rev Respir Med.* 2008;2(3):305-313.

266. Schuetz P, Leuppi JD, Tamm M, et al. Short versus conventional term glucocorticoid therapy in acute exacerbation of chronic obstructive pulmonary disease—the "REDUCE" trial. *Swiss Med Wkly.* 2010;140:w13109.

267. Pauwels RA, Buist AS, Calverley PM, Jenkins CR, Hurd SS. Global strategy for the diagnosis, management, and prevention of chronic obstructive pulmonary disease. NHLBI/WHO Global Initiative for Chronic Obstructive Lung Disease (GOLD) Workshop summary. *Am J Respir Crit Care Med.* 2001;163(5):1256-1276.

268. Burge PS, Calverley PM, Jones PW, Spencer S, Anderson JA, Maslen TK. Randomised, double blind, placebo controlled study of fluticasone propionate in patients with moderate to severe chronic obstructive pulmonary disease: the ISOLDE trial. *BMJ.* 2000;320(7245):1297-1303.

269. Cave AC, Hurst MM. The use of long acting beta-agonists, alone or in combination with inhaled corticosteroids, in chronic obstructive pulmonary disease (COPD): a risk-benefit analysis. *Pharmacol Ther.* 2011;130(2):114-143.

270. Eaton T, Fergusson W, Kolbe J, Lewis CA, West T. Short-burst oxygen therapy for COPD patients: a 6-month randomised, controlled study. *Eur Respir J.* 2006;27(4):697-704.

271. Ingadottir TS, Jonsdottir H. Technological dependency—the experience of using home ventilators and long-term oxygen therapy: patients' and families' perspective. *Scand J Caring Sci.* 2006;20(1):18-25.

272. Eaton T, Garrett JE, Young P, et al. Ambulatory oxygen improves quality of life of COPD patients: a randomised controlled study. *Eur Respir J.* 2002;20(2):306-312.

273. Abernethy AP, McDonald CF, Frith PA, et al. Effect of palliative oxygen versus room air in relief of breathlessness in patients with refractory dyspnoea: a double-blind, randomised controlled trial. *Lancet.* 2010;376(9743):784-793.

274. Uronis H, McCrory DC, Samsa G, Currow D, Abernethy A. Symptomatic oxygen for non-hypoxaemic chronic obstructive pulmonary disease. *Cochrane Database Syst Rev.* 2011(6):CD006429.

275 O'Donnell DE, Aaron S, Bourbeau J, et al. State of the Art Compendium: Canadian Thoracic Society recommendations for the management of chronic obstructive pulmonary disease. *Can Respir J.* 2004;11(Suppl B):7B-59B.

276. Abernethy AP, Currow DC, Frith P, Fazekas BS, McHugh A, Bui C. Randomised, double blind, placebo controlled crossover trial of sustained release morphine for the management of refractory dyspnoea. *BMJ.* 2003;327(7414):523-528.

277. Currow DC, McDonald C, Oaten S, et al. Once-daily opioids for chronic dyspnea: a dose increment and pharmacovigilance study. *J Pain Symptom Manage.* 2011.

278. Foral PA, Malesker MA, Huerta G, Hilleman DE. Nebulized opioids use in COPD. *Chest.* 2004;125(2):691-694.

279. Walsh TD, Rivera NI, Kaiko R. Oral morphine and respiratory function amongst hospice inpatients with advanced cancer. *Support Care Cancer.* 2003;11(12):780-784.

280. Abramson MJ, Crockett AJ, Frith PA, McDonald CF. COPDX: an update of guidelines for the management of chronic obstructive pulmonary disease with a review of recent evidence. *Med J Aust.* 2006;184(7):342-345.

281. Simon ST, Higginson IJ, Booth S, Harding R, Bausewein C. Benzodiazepines for the relief of breathlessness in advanced malignant and non-malignant diseases in adults. *Cochrane Database Syst Rev.* 2010(1):CD007354.

282. Bausewein C, Booth S, Gysels M, Higginson I. Non-pharmacological interventions for breathlessness in advanced stages of malignant and non-malignant diseases. *Cochrane Database Syst Rev.* 2008(2):CD005623.

283. Booth S, Moffat C, Burkin J, Galbraith S, Bausewein C. Nonpharmacological interventions for breathlessness. *Curr Opin Support Palliat Care.* 2011;5(2):77-86.

284. Facchiano L, Hoffman Snyder C, Nunez DE. A literature review on breathing retraining as a self-management strategy operationalized through

Rosswurm and Larrabee's evidence-based practice model. *J Am Acad Nurse Pract.* 2011;23(8):421-426.

285. Bausewein C, Booth S, Gysels M, Kuhnbach R, Higginson IJ. Effectiveness of a hand-held fan for breathlessness: a randomised phase II trial. *BMC Palliat Care.* 2010;9:22.

286. Criner GJ. Alternatives to lung transplantation: lung volume reduction for COPD. *Clin Chest Med.* 2011;32(2):379-397.

287. Nici L, Donner C, Wouters E, et al. American Thoracic Society/European Respiratory Society statement on pulmonary rehabilitation. *Am J Respir Crit Care Med.* 2006;173(12):1390-1413.

288. Bourbeau J, Julien M, Maltais F, et al. Reduction of hospital utilization in patients with chronic obstructive pulmonary disease: a disease-specific self-management intervention. *Arch Intern Med.* 2003;163(5):585-591.

289. Lacasse Y, Brosseau L, Milne S, et al. Pulmonary rehabilitation for chronic obstructive pulmonary disease. *Cochrane Database Syst Rev.* 2002;(3):CD003793.

290. Effing T, Zielhuis G, Kerstjens H, van der Valk P, van der Palen J. Community based physiotherapeutic exercise in COPD self-management: a randomised controlled trial. *Respir Med.* 2011;105(3):418-426.

291. Spencer LM, Alison JA, McKeough ZJ. Maintaining benefits following pulmonary rehabilitation: a randomised controlled trial. *Eur Respir J.* 2010;35(3):571-577.

292. Bourbeau J, Nault D, Dang-Tan T. Self-management and behaviour modification in COPD. *Patient Educ Couns.* 2004;52(3):271-277.

293. Curtis JR, Wenrich MD, Carline JD, Shannon SE, Ambrozy DM, Ramsey PG. Patients' perspectives on physician skill in end-of-life care: differences between patients with COPD, cancer, and AIDS. *Chest.* 2002;122(1):356-362.

294. Effing T, Monninkhof EM, van der Valk PD, et al. Self-management education for patients with chronic obstructive pulmonary disease. *Cochrane Database Syst Rev.* 2007;(4):CD002990.

295. Janssen DJ, Spruit MA, Alsemgeest TP, Does JD, Schols JM, Wouters EF. A patient-centred interdisciplinary palliative care programme for end-stage chronic respiratory diseases. *Int J Palliat Nurs.* 2010;16(4):189-194.

296. Bredin M, Corner J, Krishnasamy M, Plant H, Bailey C, A'Hern R. Multicentre randomised controlled trial of nursing intervention for breathlessness in patients with lung cancer. *BMJ.* 1999;318(7188):901-904.

297. Booth S, Farquhar M, Gysels M, Bausewein C, Higginson IJ. The impact of a breathlessness intervention service (BIS) on the lives of patients with intractable dyspnea: a qualitative phase 1 study. *Palliat Support Care.* 2006;4(3):287-293.

298. Schwartzstein RM, Lahive K, Pope A, Weinberger SE, Weiss JW. Cold facial stimulation reduces breathlessness induced in normal subjects. *Am Rev Respir Dis.* 1987;136(1):58-61.

299. Keenan SP, Sinuff T, Cook DJ, Hill NS. Which patients with acute exacerbation of chronic obstructive pulmonary disease benefit from noninvasive positive-pressure ventilation? A systematic review of the literature. *Ann Intern Med.* 2003;138(11):861-870.

300. Benhamou D, Girault C, Faure C, Portier F, Muir JF. Nasal mask ventilation in acute respiratory failure. Experience in elderly patients. *Chest.* 1992;102(3):912-917.

301. Meduri GU, Fox RC, Abou-Shala N, Leeper KV, Wunderink RG. Noninvasive mechanical ventilation via face mask in patients with acute respiratory failure who refused endotracheal intubation. *Crit Care Med.* 1994;22(10):1584-1590.

302. Elliott MW. Non-invasive ventilation: established and expanding roles. *Clin Med.* 2011;11(2):150-153.

303. Benditt JO. Noninvasive ventilation at the end of life. *Respir Care.* 2000;45(11):1376-1381.

304. Curtis JR, Cook DJ, Sinuff T, et al. Noninvasive positive pressure ventilation in critical and palliative care settings: understanding the goals of therapy. *Crit Care Med.* 2007;35(3):932-939.

305. Gardiner C, Gott M, Payne S, et al. Exploring the care needs of patients with advanced COPD: an overview of the literature. *Respir Med.* 2010;104(2):159-165.

306. Curtis JR, Engelberg RA, Nielsen EL, Au DH, Patrick DL. Patient-physician communication about end-of-life care for patients with severe COPD. *Eur Respir J.* 2004;24(2):200-205.

307. Heyland DK, Dodek P, Rocker G, et al. What matters most in end-of-life care: perceptions of seriously ill patients and their family members. *CMAJ.* 2006;174(5):627-633.

308. Heyland DK, Groll D, Rocker G, et al. End-of-life care in acute care hospitals in Canada: a quality finish? *J Palliat Care*. 2005;21(3):142-150.

309. Seamark DA, Seamark CJ, Halpin DM. Palliative care in chronic obstructive pulmonary disease: a review for clinicians. *J R Soc Med*. May 2007;100(5):225-233.

310. Mikkelsen RL, Middelboe T, Pisinger C, Stage KB. Anxiety and depression in patients with chronic obstructive pulmonary disease (COPD). A review. *Nord J Psychiatry*. 2004;58(1):65-70.

311. van Ede L, Yzermans CJ, Brouwer HJ. Prevalence of depression in patients with chronic obstructive pulmonary disease: a systematic review. *Thorax*. 1999;54(8):688-692.

312. Schneider C, Jick SS, Bothner U, Meier CR. COPD and the risk of depression. *Chest*. 2010;137(2):341-347.

313. Kim HF, Kunik ME, Molinari VA, et al. Functional impairment in COPD patients: the impact of anxiety and depression. *Psychosomatics*. 2000;41(6):465-471.

314. Balcells E, Gea J, Ferrer J, et al. Factors affecting the relationship between psychological status and quality of life in COPD patients. *Health Qual Life Outcomes*. 2010;8:108.

315. Ferrer M, Alonso J, Morera J, et al. Chronic obstructive pulmonary disease stage and health-related quality of life. The Quality of Life of Chronic Obstructive Pulmonary Disease Study Group. *Ann Intern Med*. 1997;127(12):1072-1079.

316. Lacasse Y, Rousseau L, Maltais F. Prevalence of depressive symptoms and depression in patients with severe oxygen-dependent chronic obstructive pulmonary disease. *J Cardiopulm Rehabil*. 2001;21(2):80-86.

317. McSweeney AJ, Grant I, Heaton RK, Adams KM, Timms RM. Life quality of patients with chronic obstructive pulmonary disease. *Arch Intern Med*. 1982;142(3):473-478.

318. Di Marco F, Verga M, Reggente M, et al. Anxiety and depression in COPD patients: the roles of gender and disease severity. *Respir Med*. 2006;100(10):1767-1774.

319. Gudmundsson G, Gislason T, Janson C, et al. Depression, anxiety and health status after hospitalisation for COPD: a multicentre study in the Nordic countries. *Respir Med*. 2006;100(1):87-93.

320. Borson S, McDonald GJ, Gayle T, Deffebach M, Lakshminarayan S, VanTuinen C. Improvement in mood, physical symptoms, and function with nortriptyline for depression in patients with chronic obstructive pulmonary disease. *Psychosomatics*. 1992;33(2):190-201.

321. Smoller JW, Pollack MH, Otto MW, Rosenbaum JF, Kradin RL. Panic anxiety, dyspnea, and respiratory disease. Theoretical and clinical considerations. *Am J Respir Crit Care Med*. 1996;154(1):6-17.

322. Eiser N, West C, Evans S, Jeffers A, Quirk F. Effects of psychotherapy in moderately severe COPD: a pilot study. *Eur Respir J*. 1997;10(7):1581-1584.

323. Runo JR, Ely EW. Treating dyspnea in a patient with advanced chronic obstructive pulmonary disease. *West J Med*. 2001;175(3):197-201.

324. Manning HL. Dyspnea treatment. *Respir Care*. 2000;45(11):1342-1350; discussion 1350-1344.

325. Hynninen MJ, Bjerke N, Pallesen S, Bakke PS, Nordhus IH. A randomized controlled trial of cognitive behavioral therapy for anxiety and depression in COPD. *Respir Med*. 2010;104(7):986-994.

326. Eisner MD, Blanc PD, Yelin EH, et al. Influence of anxiety on health outcomes in COPD. *Thorax*. 2010;65(3):229-234.

327. Stage KB, Middelboe T, Pisinger C. Depression and chronic obstructive pulmonary disease. Impact on survival. *Acta Psychiatr Scand*. 2005;111(4):320-323.

328. de Voogd JN, Wempe JB, Koeter GH, et al. Depressive symptoms as predictors of mortality in patients with COPD. *Chest*. 2009;135(3):619-625.

329. Stapleton RD, Nielsen EL, Engelberg RA, Patrick DL, Curtis JR. Association of depression and life-sustaining treatment preferences in patients with COPD. *Chest*. 2005;127(1):328-334.

330. Reinke LF, Slatore CG, Udris EM, Moss BR, Johnson EA, Au DH. The association of depression and preferences for life-sustaining treatments in veterans with chronic obstructive pulmonary disease. *J Pain Symptom Manage*. 2011;41(2):402-411.

331. Garuti G, Cilione C, Dell'Orso D, et al. Impact of comprehensive pulmonary rehabilitation on anxiety and depression in hospitalized COPD patients. *Monaldi Arch Chest Dis*. 2003;59(1):56-61.

332. Booth S, Silvester S, Todd C. Breathlessness in cancer and chronic obstructive pulmonary disease: using a qualitative approach to describe the experience of patients and carers. *Palliat Support Care*. 2003;1(4):337-344.

333. Heffner JE, Fahy B, Hilling L, Barbieri C. Attitudes regarding advance directives among patients in pulmonary rehabilitation. *Am J Respir Crit Care Med.* 1996;154(6 Pt 1):1735-1740.

334. Janssen DJ, Spruit MA, Schols JM, Wouters EF. A call for high-quality advance care planning in outpatients with severe COPD or chronic heart failure. *Chest.* May 2011;139(5):1081-1088.

335. Reinke LF, Slatore CG, Uman J, et al. Patient-clinician communication about end-of-life care topics: is anyone talking to patients with chronic obstructive pulmonary disease? *J Palliat Med.* 2011;14(8):923-928.

336. Johnston SC, Pfeifer MP, McNutt R. The discussion about advance directives. Patient and physician opinions regarding when and how it should be conducted. End of Life Study Group. *Arch Intern Med.* 1995;155(10):1025-1030.

337. Gott M, Gardiner C, Small N, et al. Barriers to advance care planning in chronic obstructive pulmonary disease. *Palliat Med.* 2009;23(7):642-648.

338. Janssen DJ, Engelberg RA, Wouters EF, Curtis JR. Advance care planning for patients with COPD: Past, present and future. *Patient Educ Couns.* 2011.

339. Wilson KG, Aaron SD, Vandemheen KL, et al. Evaluation of a decision aid for making choices about intubation and mechanical ventilation in chronic obstructive pulmonary disease. *Patient Educ Couns.* 2005;57(1):88-95.

340. Dales RE, O'Connor A, Hebert P, Sullivan K, McKim D, Llewellyn-Thomas H. Intubation and mechanical ventilation for COPD: development of an instrument to elicit patient preferences. *Chest.* 1999;116(3):792-800.

341. National Hospice and Palliative Care Organization. NHPCO facts and figures: hospice care in America [National Hospice and Palliative Care Organization website]. Available at: www.nhpco.org/files/public/Statistics_Research/Hospice_Facts_Figures_Oct-2010.pdf. Accessed April 7, 2011.

342. Fox E, Landrum-McNiff K, Zhong Z, Dawson NV, Wu AW, Lynn J. Evaluation of prognostic criteria for determining hospice eligibility in patients with advanced lung, heart, or liver disease. SUPPORT Investigators. Study to Understand Prognoses and Preferences for Outcomes and Risks of Treatments. *JAMA.* 1999;282(17):1638-1645.

343. Ehman JW, Ott BB, Short TH, Ciampa RC, Hansen-Flaschen J. Do patients want physicians to inquire about their spiritual or religious beliefs if they become gravely ill? *Arch Intern Med.* 1999;159(15):1803-1806.

344. Saguil A, Fitzpatrick AL, Clark G. Is evidence able to persuade physicians to discuss spirituality with patients? *J Relig Health.* 2011;50(2):289-299.

345. Sprung CL, Cohen SL, Sjokvist P, et al. End-of-life practices in European intensive care units: the Ethicus Study. *JAMA.* 2003;290(6):790-797.

346. Post SG, Puchalski CM, Larson DB. Physicians and patient spirituality: professional boundaries, competency, and ethics. *Ann Intern Med.* 2000;132(7):578-583.

347. Lo B, Ruston D, Kates LW, et al. Discussing religious and spiritual issues at the end of life: a practical guide for physicians. *JAMA.* 2002;287(6):749-754.

348. Gijsberts MJ, Echteld MA, van der Steen JT, et al. Spirituality at the end of life: conceptualization of measurable aspects-a systematic review. *J Palliat Med.* 2011;14(7):852-863.

349. Albers G, Echteld MA, de Vet HC, Onwuteaka-Philipsen BD, van der Linden MH, Deliens L. Content and spiritual items of quality-of-life instruments appropriate for use in palliative care: a review. *J Pain Symptom Manage.* 2010;40(2):290-300.

350. Lindqvist G, Hallberg LR. 'Feelings of guilt due to self-inflicted disease': a grounded theory of suffering from chronic obstructive pulmonary disease (COPD). *J Health Psychol.* 2010;15(3):456-466.

351. Meador KG. Spiritual care at the end of life: what is it and who does it? *N C Med J.* 2004;65(4):226-228.

352. Curtis JR, Engelberg RA, Wenrich MD, Au DH. Communication about palliative care for patients with chronic obstructive pulmonary disease. *J Palliat Care.* 2005;21(3):157-164.

353. Puchalski CM, Lunsford B, Harris MH, Miller RT. Interdisciplinary spiritual care for seriously ill and dying patients: a collaborative model. *Cancer J.* 2006;12(5):398-416.

354. Steinhauser KE, Voils CI, Clipp EC, Bosworth HB, Christakis NA, Tulsky JA. "Are you at peace?" One item to probe spiritual concerns at the end of life. *Arch Intern Med.* 2006;166(1):101-105.

355. Green MR, Emery CF, Kozora E, Diaz PT, Make BJ. Religious and spiritual coping and quality of life among patients with emphysema in the National Emphysema Treatment Trial. *Respir Care.* 2011;56(10):1514-1521.

356. Puchalski CM, Kilpatrick SD, McCullough ME, Larson DB. A systematic review of spiritual and religious variables in Palliative Medicine, American Journal of Hospice and Palliative Care, Hospice Journal, Journal of Palliative Care, and Journal of Pain and Symptom Management. *Palliat Support Care*. 2003;1(1):7-13.

357. Fitchett G, Lyndes KA, Cadge W, Berlinger N, Flanagan E, Misasi J. The role of professional chaplains on pediatric palliative care teams: perspectives from physicians and chaplains. *J Palliat Med*. 2011;14(6):704-707.

358. Steinhauser KE, Christakis NA, Clipp EC, et al. Preparing for the end of life: preferences of patients, families, physicians, and other care providers. *J Pain Symptom Manage*. 2001;22(3):727-737.

359. Emanuel EJ, Fairclough DL, Slutsman J, Emanuel LL. Understanding economic and other burdens of terminal illness: the experience of patients and their caregivers. *Ann Intern Med*. 2000;132(6):451-459.

360. Grunfeld E, Coyle D, Whelan T, et al. Family caregiver burden: results of a longitudinal study of breast cancer patients and their principal caregivers. *CMAJ*. 2004;170(12):1795-1801.

361. Nijboer C, Triemstra M, Tempelaar R, Mulder M, Sanderman R, van den Bos GA. Patterns of caregiver experiences among partners of cancer patients. *Gerontologist*. 2000;40(6):738-746.

362. Song JI, Shin DW, Choi JY, et al. Quality of life and mental health in the bereaved family members of patients with terminal cancer. *Psycho-oncology*. Aug 7 2011.

363. Higginson IJ, Finlay IG, Goodwin DM, et al. Is there evidence that palliative care teams alter end-of-life experiences of patients and their caregivers? *J Pain Symptom Manage*. 2003;25(2):150-168.

364. Williams AL, McCorkle R. Cancer family caregivers during the palliative, hospice, and bereavement phases: a review of the descriptive psychosocial literature. *Palliat Support Care*. 2011;9(3):315-325.

365. Harding R, Higginson IJ. What is the best way to help caregivers in cancer and palliative care? A systematic literature review of interventions and their effectiveness. *Palliat Med*. 2003;17(1):63-74.

366. O'Hara RE, Hull JG, Lyons KD, et al. Impact on caregiver burden of a patient-focused palliative care intervention for patients with advanced cancer. *Palliat Support Care*. 2010;8(4):395-404.

367. Wakabayashi R, Motegi T, Yamada K, Ishii T, Gemma A, Kida K. Presence of in-home caregiver and health outcomes of older adults with chronic obstructive pulmonary disease. *J Am Geriatr Soc*. 2011;59(1):44-49.

368. Bailey PH. Death stories: acute exacerbations of chronic obstructive pulmonary disease. *Qual Health Res*. 2001;11(3):322-338.

369. Seamark DA, Blake SD, Seamark CJ, Halpin DM. Living with severe chronic obstructive pulmonary disease (COPD): perceptions of patients and their carers. An interpretative phenomenological analysis. *Palliat Med*. 2004;18(7):619-625.

370. Cannuscio CC, Jones C, Kawachi I, Colditz GA, Berkman L, Rimm E. Reverberations of family illness: a longitudinal assessment of informal caregiving and mental health status in the Nurses' Health Study. *Am J Public Health*. 2002;92(8):1305-1311.

371. Bergs D. "The Hidden Client"--women caring for husbands with COPD: their experience of quality of life. *J Clin Nurs*. 2002;11(5):613-621.

372. Garlo K, O'Leary JR, Van Ness PH, Fried TR. Burden in caregivers of older adults with advanced illness. *J Am Geriatr Soc*. 2010;58(12):2315-2322.

373. Skilbeck J, Mott L, Page H, Smith D, Hjelmeland-Ahmedzai S, Clark D. Palliative care in chronic obstructive airways disease: a needs assessment. *Palliat Med*. 1998;12(4):245-254.

374. Gries CJ, Engelberg RA, Kross EK, et al. Predictors of symptoms of posttraumatic stress and depression in family members after patient death in the ICU. *Chest*. 2010;137(2):280-287.

375. Nicolson P, Anderson P. Quality of life, distress and self-esteem: a focus group study of people with chronic bronchitis. *Br J Health Psychol*. 2003;8(Pt 3):251-270.

376. Monninkhof E, van der Aa M, van der Valk P, et al. A qualitative evaluation of a comprehensive self-management programme for COPD patients: effectiveness from the patients' perspective. *Patient Educ Couns*. 2004;55(2):177-184.

377. Engstrom CP, Persson LO, Larsson S, Sullivan M. Health-related quality of life in COPD: why both disease-specific and generic measures should be used. *Eur Respir J*. 2001;18(1):69-76.

378. Hughes SL, Weaver FM, Giobbie-Hurder A, et al. Effectiveness of team-managed home-based primary care: a randomized multicenter trial. *JAMA*. 2000;284(22):2877-2885.

379. Pinnock H, Huby G, Tierney A, et al. Is multidisciplinary teamwork the key? A qualitative study of the development of respiratory services in the UK. *J R Soc Med*. 2009;102(9):378-390.

380. Kuzma AM, Meli Y, Meldrum C, et al. Multidisciplinary care of the patient with chronic obstructive pulmonary disease. *Proceedings of the American Thoracic Society*. 2008;5(4):567-571.

381. Hopp FP, Thornton N, Martin L. The lived experience of heart failure at the end of life: a systematic literature review. *Health Soc Work*. 2010;35(2):109-117.

382. Hunt SA, Abraham WT, Chin MH, et al. ACC/AHA 2005 Guideline Update for the Diagnosis and Management of Chronic Heart Failure in the Adult: a report of the American College of Cardiology/American Heart Association Task Force on Practice Guidelines (Writing Committee to Update the 2001 Guidelines for the Evaluation and Management of Heart Failure): developed in collaboration with the American College of Chest Physicians and the International Society for Heart and Lung Transplantation: endorsed by the Heart Rhythm Society. *Circulation*. Sep 20 2005;112(12):e154-235.

383. Hunt SA, Abraham WT, Chin MH, et al. 2009 focused update incorporated into the ACC/AHA 2005 Guidelines for the Diagnosis and Management of Heart Failure in Adults: a report of the American College of Cardiology Foundation/American Heart Association Task Force on Practice Guidelines: developed in collaboration with the International Society for Heart and Lung Transplantation. *Circulation*. 2009;119(14):e391-479.

384. Lloyd-Jones D, Adams RJ, Brown TM, et al. Heart disease and stroke statistics--2010 update: a report from the American Heart Association. *Circulation*. 2010;121(7):e46-e215.

385. Roger VL. The heart failure epidemic. *Int J Environ Res Public Health*. Apr 2010;7(4):1807-1830.

386. Miller LW, Lietz K. Candidate selection for long-term left ventricular assist device therapy for refractory heart failure. *J Heart Lung Transplant*. 2006;25(7):756-764.

387. Bekelman DB, Rumsfeld JS, Havranek EP, et al. Symptom burden, depression, and spiritual well-being: a comparison of heart failure and advanced cancer patients. *J Gen Intern Med*. 2009;24(5):592-598.

388. Goodlin SJ, Quill TE, Arnold RM. Communication and decision-making about prognosis in heart failure care. *J Card Fail*. 2008;14(2):106-113.

389. Goodlin SJ. Palliative care in congestive heart failure. *J Am Coll Cardiol*. 2009;54(5):386-396.

390. Jessup M, Abraham WT, Casey DE, et al. 2009 focused update: ACCF/AHA Guidelines for the Diagnosis and Management of Heart Failure in Adults: a report of the American College of Cardiology Foundation/American Heart Association Task Force on Practice Guidelines: developed in collaboration with the International Society for Heart and Lung Transplantation. *Circulation*. 2009;119(14):1977-2016.

391. McCarthy M, Lay M, Addington-Hall J. Dying from heart disease. *J R Coll Physicians Lond*. 1996;30(4):325-328.

392. Gibbs LM, Addington-Hall J, Gibbs JS. Dying from heart failure: lessons from palliative care. Many patients would benefit from palliative care at the end of their lives. *BMJ*. 1998;317(7164):961-962.

393. Hauptman PJ, Havranek EP. Integrating palliative care into heart failure care. *Arch Intern Med*. 2005;165(4):374-378.

394. Goodlin SJ, Hauptman PJ, Arnold R, et al. Consensus statement: Palliative and supportive care in advanced heart failure. *J Card Fail*. 2004;10(3):200-209.

395. Roger VL, Go AS, Lloyd-Jones DM, et al. Heart disease and stroke statistics--2011 update: a report from the American Heart Association. *Circulation*. 2011;123(4):e18-e209.

396. Medicare coverage expanded. New York Times. January 28, 2005. Available at: http://query.nytimes.com/gst/fullpage.html?res=9F05E2DE143BF93BA15752C0A9639C8B63&scp=1&sq=Medicare+coverage+expanded&st=nyt. Accessed February 27, 2012.

397. Nichol G, Kaul P, Huszti E, Bridges JF. Cost-effectiveness of cardiac resynchronization therapy in patients with symptomatic heart failure. *Ann Intern Med*. 2004;141(5):343-351.

398. Digiorgi PL, Reel MS, Thornton B, Burton E, Naka Y, Oz MC. Heart transplant and left ventricular assist device costs. *J Heart Lung Transplant*. 2005;24(2):200-204.

399. Slaughter MS, Bostic R, Tong K, Russo M, Rogers JG. Temporal changes in hospital costs for left ventricular assist device implantation. *J Card Surg.* 2011;26(5):535-541.

400. Levenson JW, McCarthy EP, Lynn J, Davis RB, Phillips RS. The last six months of life for patients with congestive heart failure. *J Am Geriatr Soc.* 2000;48(5 Suppl):S101-109.

401. Packer DL, Prutkin JM, Hellkamp AS, et al. Impact of implantable cardioverter-defibrillator, amiodarone, and placebo on the mode of death in stable patients with heart failure: analysis from the sudden cardiac death in heart failure trial. *Circulation.* 2009;120(22):2170-2176.

402. U.S. Food and Drug Administration. FDA approves left ventricular assist system for severe heart failure patients. January 20, 2010. Available at: www.fda.gov/NewsEvents/Newsroom/PressAnnouncements/ucm198172.htm. Accessed August 17, 2011.

403. Goldstein NE, Lynn J. Trajectory of end-stage heart failure: the influence of technology and implications for policy change. *Perspect Biol Med.* 2006;49(1):10-18.

404. Packer M. Lack of relation between ventricular arrhythmias and sudden death in patients with chronic heart failure. *Circulation.* 1992;85(1 Suppl):I50-56.

405. Teuteberg JJ, Teuteberg WG. Course to death in heart failure. In: Beattie J, Goodlin SJ, eds. *Supportive Care of the Cardiac Patient.* New York, NY: Oxford University Press; 2006.

406. Yancy CW, Lopatin M, Stevenson LW, De Marco T, Fonarow GC. Clinical presentation, management, and in-hospital outcomes of patients admitted with acute decompensated heart failure with preserved systolic function: a report from the Acute Decompensated Heart Failure National Registry (ADHERE) Database. *J Am Coll Cardiol.* 2006;47(1):76-84.

407. Borlaug BA, Redfield MM. Diastolic and systolic heart failure are distinct phenotypes within the heart failure spectrum. *Circulation.* 2011;123(18):2006-2013.

408. Wood P, Piran S, Liu PP. Diastolic heart failure: progress, treatment challenges, and prevention. *Can J Cardiol.* 2011;27(3):302-310.

409. Zile MR, Gaasch WH, Anand IS, et al. Mode of death in patients with heart failure and a preserved ejection fraction: results from the Irbesartan in Heart Failure With Preserved Ejection Fraction Study (I-Preserve) trial. *Circulation.* 2010;121(12):1393-1405.

410. Rogers JG, Butler J, Lansman SL, et al. Chronic mechanical circulatory support for inotrope-dependent heart failure patients who are not transplant candidates: results of the INTrEPID Trial. *J Am Coll Cardiol.* 2007;50(8):741-747.

411. Slaughter MS, Rogers JG, Milano CA, et al. Advanced heart failure treated with continuous-flow left ventricular assist device. *N Engl J Med.* 2009;361(23):2241-2251.

412. Fang JC. Rise of the machines—left ventricular assist devices as permanent therapy for advanced heart failure. *N Engl J Med.* 2009;361(23):2282-2285.

413. Nohria A, Lewis E, Stevenson LW. Medical management of advanced heart failure. *JAMA.* 2002;287(5):628-640.

414. Marti C, Cole R, Kalogeropoulos A, Georgiopoulou V, Butler J. Medical therapy for acute decompensated heart failure: what recent clinical trials have taught us about diuretics and vasodilators. *Curr Heart Fail Rep.* 2011.

415. O'Connor CM, Gattis WA, Uretsky BF, et al. Continuous intravenous dobutamine is associated with an increased risk of death in patients with advanced heart failure: insights from the Flolan International Randomized Survival Trial (FIRST). *Am Heart J.* 1999;138(1):78-86.

416. Lee DS, Stukel TA, Austin PC, et al. Improved outcomes with early collaborative care of ambulatory heart failure patients discharged from the emergency department. *Circulation.* 2010;122(18):1806-1814.

417. Zacharias H, Raw J, Nunn A, Parsons S, Johnson M. Is there a role for subcutaneous furosemide in the community and hospice management of end-stage heart failure? *Palliat Med.* 2011.

418. O'Connor CM, Starling RC, Hernandez AF, et al. Effect of nesiritide in patients with acute decompensated heart failure. *N Engl J Med.* 2011;365(1):32-43.

419. Gorodeski EZ, Chu EC, Reese JR, Shishehbor MH, Hsich E, Starling RC. Prognosis on chronic dobutamine or milrinone infusions for stage D heart failure. *Circ Heart Fail.* 2009;2(4):320-324.

420. Bhattacharya S, Abebe K, Simon M, Saba S, Adelstein E. Role of cardiac resynchronization in end-stage heart failure patients requiring inotrope therapy. *J Card Fail.* 2010;16(12):931-937.

421. Villet OM, Siltanen A, Patila T, et al. Advances in cell transplantation therapy for diseased myocardium. *Stem Cells Int.* 2011;2011:679171.

422. Maçiver J, Rao V, Ross HJ. Quality of life for patients supported on a left ventricular assist device. *Expert Rev Med Devices.* 2011;8(3):325-337.

423. Bax JJ, Abraham T, Barold SS, et al. Cardiac resynchronization therapy: Part 1—issues before device implantation. *J Am Coll Cardiol.* 2005;46(12):2153-2167.

424. Lamont EB, Christakis NA. Prognostic disclosure to patients with cancer near the end of life. *Ann Intern Med.* 2001;134(12):1096-1105.

425. Eichorn EJ. Prognosis determination in heart failure. *Am J Med.* 2001;110(suppl 7A):14S-35S.

426. Levy WC, Mozaffarian D, Linker DT, et al. The Seattle Heart Failure Model: prediction of survival in heart failure. *Circulation.* 2006;113(11):1424-1433.

427. Cleland JG, Daubert JC, Erdmann E, et al. The effect of cardiac resynchronization on morbidity and mortality in heart failure. *N Engl J Med.* 2005;352(15):1539-1549.

428. Bristow MR, Saxon LA, Boehmer J, et al. Cardiac-resynchronization therapy with or without an implantable defibrillator in advanced chronic heart failure. *N Engl J Med.* 2004;350(21):2140-2150.

429. Rose EA, Gelijns AC, Moskowitz AJ, et al. Long-term use of a left ventricular assist device for end-stage heart failure. *N Engl J Med.* 2001;345(20):1435-1443.

430. Hershberger RE, Nauman D, Walker TL, Dutton D, Burgess D. Care processes and clinical outcomes of continuous outpatient support with inotropes (COSI) in patients with refractory endstage heart failure. *J Card Fail.* 2003;9(3):180-187.

431. Lewis EF, Johnson PA, Johnson W, Collins C, Griffin L, Stevenson LW. Preferences for quality of life or survival expressed by patients with heart failure. *J Heart Lung Transplant.* 2001;20(9):1016-1024.

432. Stanek EJ, Oates MB, McGhan WF, Denofrio D, Loh E. Preferences for treatment outcomes in patients with heart failure: symptoms versus survival. *J Card Fail.* 2000;6(3):225-232.

433. Krumholz HM, Phillips RS, Hamel MB, et al. Resuscitation preferences among patients with severe congestive heart failure: results from the SUPPORT project. Study to Understand Prognoses and Preferences for Outcomes and Risks of Treatments. *Circulation.* 1998;98(7):648-655.

434. Wachter RM, Luce JM, Hearst N, Lo B. Decisions about resuscitation: inequities among patients with different diseases but similar prognoses. *Ann Intern Med.* 1989;111(6):525-532.

435. McCarthy M, Hall JA, Ley M. Communication and choice in dying from heart disease. *J R Soc Med.* 1997;90(3):128-131.

436. Swetz KM, Freeman MR, AbouEzzeddine OF, et al. Palliative medicine consultation for preparedness planning in patients receiving left ventricular assist devices as destination therapy. *Mayo Clin Proc.* 2011;86(6):493-500.

437. Scott LD. Caregiving and care receiving among a technologically dependent heart failure population. *ANS Adv Nurs Sci.* 2000;23(2):82-97.

438. Hochgerner M, Fruhwald FM, Strohscheer I. Opioids for symptomatic therapy of dyspnoea in patients with advanced chronic heart failure—is there evidence? *Wien Med Wochenschr.* 2009;159(23-24):577-582.

439. Davidson PM, Johnson MJ. Update on the role of palliative oxygen. *Curr Opin Support Palliat Care.* 2011;5(2):87-91.

440. Goebel JR, Doering LV, Shugarman LR, et al. Heart failure: the hidden problem of pain. *J Pain Symptom Manage.* 2009;38(5):698-707.

441. Shapiro PA. Treatment of depression in patients with congestive heart failure. *Heart Fail Rev.* 2009;14(1):7-12.

442. Ghali JK, Anand IS, Abraham WT, et al. Randomized double-blind trial of darbepoetin alfa in patients with symptomatic heart failure and anemia. *Circulation.* 2008;117(4):526-535.

443. Iellamo F, Volterrani M, Caminiti G, et al. Testosterone therapy in women with chronic heart failure: a pilot double-blind, randomized, placebo-controlled study. *J Am Coll Cardiol.* 2010;56(16):1310-1316.

444. Teuteberg JJ, Lewis EF, Nohria A, et al. Characteristics of patients who die with heart failure and a low ejection fraction in the new millennium. *J Card Fail.* 2006;12(1):47-53

445. Petrucci RJ, Benish LA, Carrow BL, et al. Ethical considerations for ventricular assist device support: a 10-point model. *Asaio J.* 2011;57(4):268-273.

446. Kramer DB, Ottenberg AL, Mueller PS. Management of cardiac electrical implantable devices in patients nearing the end of life or requesting withdrawal of therapy: review of the Heart Rhythm Society 2010 consensus statement. *Pol Arch Med Wewn*. 2010;120(12):497-502.

447. Goldstein NE, Lampert R, Bradley E, Lynn J, Krumholz HM. Management of implantable cardioverter defibrillators in end-of-life care. *Ann Intern Med*. 2004;141(11):835-838.

448. Bramstedt KA, Wenger NS. When withdrawal of life-sustaining care does more than allow death to take its course: the dilemma of left ventricular assist devices. *J Heart Lung Transplant*. 2001;20(5):544-548.

449. Brush S, Budge D, Alharethi R, et al. End-of-life decision making and implementation in recipients of a destination left ventricular assist device. *J Heart Lung Transplant*. 2010;29(12):1337-1341.

450. Green E, Gardiner C, Gott M, Ingleton C. Exploring the extent of communication surrounding transitions to palliative care in heart failure: the perspectives of health care professionals. *J Palliat Care*. 2011;27(2):107-116.

451. Gibbs JS, McCoy AS, Gibbs LM, Rogers AE, Addington-Hall JM. Living with and dying from heart failure: the role of palliative care. *Heart*. 2002;88 Suppl 2:ii36-39.

452. US Mortality Public Use Data Tape 2002, National Center for Health Statistics, Centers for Disease Control and Prevention. 2004.

453. Setoguchi S, Glynn RJ, Stedman M, Flavell CM, Levin R, Stevenson LW. Hospice, opiates, and acute care service use among the elderly before death from heart failure or cancer. *Am Heart J*. 2010;160(1):139-144.

454. National Hospice and Palliative Care Organization. 2010 Facts and Figures [National Hospice and Palliative Care Organization website]. Available at: www.nhpco.org/files/public/statistics_research/hospice_facts_figures_oct-2010.pdf. Accessed February 27, 2012.

455. Zambroski CH, Moser DK, Roser LP, Heo S, Chung ML. Patients with heart failure who die in hospice. *Am Heart J*. 2005;149(3):558-564.

456. Bain KT, Maxwell TL, Strassels SA, Whellan DJ. Hospice use among patients with heart failure. *Am Heart J*. Jul 2009;158(1):118-125.

457. Reisfield GM, Wilson GR. Fast Facts and Concepts #143: prognostication in heart failure. Available at: http://www.eperc.mcw.edu/FileLibrary/User/jrehm/fastfactpdfs/Concept143.pdf. Accessed February 27, 2012.

458. Pressler SJ, Gradus-Pizlo I, Chubinski SD, et al. Family caregiver outcomes in heart failure. *Am J Crit Care*. 2009;18(2):149-159.

459. Dracup K, Evangelista LS, Doering L, Tullman D, Moser DK, Hamilton M. Emotional well-being in spouses of patients with advanced heart failure. *Heart Lung*. 2004;33(6):354-361.

460. Small N, Barnes S, Gott M, et al. Dying, death and bereavement: a qualitative study of the views of carers of people with heart failure in the UK. *BMC Palliat Care*. 2009;8:6.

Index

BODE (body mass, air flow obstruction, dyspnea, exercise) index, 35, 38
body mass index (BMI)
    dementia and, 14
    opioid doses and, 46
breathlessness intervention service (BIS), 49
Brief Carrol Depression Rating Scale, 17
bronchoconstriction, 43
bronchodilators, 42–43, 46–47
bumetanide, side effects, 66t
bupropion, for depression, 76

C

caffeine, 20, 21t
calcium channel blockers, 68
candesartan, side effects, 66t
captopril, side effects, 66t
carbamezapine
    dosage, 23t
    for agitation, 21, 23t
    side effects, 23t
cardiac glycosides, 66t
cardiac resynchronization therapy (CRT), 59, 69t, 72
cardiac transplantation, 59, 64–65
caregivers. see also families
    bereavement support, 32, 83
    demands on, 55–56
    information for, 53
    issues related to, 31–32
    of heart failure patients, 82–83
    patient pain experience and, 16–17
carvedilol, side effects, 66t
case managers, roles for, 82–83
chaplains, roles for, 54
Checklist of Nonverbal Pain Indicators (CNPI), 16
chest tightness, dyspnea and, 37
cholinesterase inhibitors, 6
    anorexia and, 26
    for agitation, 21, 23t
    for dementia, 7–8
    side effects, 8
chronic obstructive pulmonary disease (COPD), 35-56
    acute exacerbations, 43
    AD and, 3

chronic obstructive pulmonary disease (COPD) (cont.)
    case studies, 35–36, 39–40, 44–45, 50–51, 56
    communication in, 53
    comorbidities, 39
    disease trajectory, 36t, 37–39, 51
    epidemiology, 35–37
    management of, 41–49, 41f
    palliative care needs, 51–52
    symptom control, 40–49
    systemic manifestations, 39
chronic renal insufficiency, 78
citalopram
    dosage, 23t
    for agitation, 23t
    side effects, 23t
clonazepam, 70, 77
cognitive therapy, in COPD, 52
cognitive training, 10
Cohen-Mansfield Agitation Inventory, 20
communication
    about referrals to hospice, 79–80
    barriers to, 38
    end-of-life decision making and, 53
    hope and, 14–15
    with heart failure patients, 72–73
congestive heart failure (CHF), 57–83. see also heart failure
    caregiver issues, 82–83
    case study, 58, 62–63, 70–71, 74–75, 82
    definition of, 57–59
    dementia and, 14
    diagnostic criteria, 57–59
    disease trajectory, 63–68
    end-stage issues, 77–79
    epidemiology, 59–60
    incidence, 60–62
    invasive therapies, 68
    management of, 63–68
    prevalence, 60–62
    symptom management, 75–77
constipation
    anorexia and, 28
    opioids and, 45
    treatment, 21t

spiritual issues (*cont.*)
    illness-related distress, 54–55
    in COPD, 54–55
    well-being and, 60
spirometry, results on, 40
spironolactone, side effects, 66*t*
stem cell transplants, 68
Study to Understand Prognoses and Preferences for
  Outcomes and Risks of Treatment (SUPPORT), 37, 62
subcortical infarcts, 2
swallowing difficulties, 25

T

tachycardia, resting, 51, 54
tau protein, 2
testosterone supplementation, 77
theophylline
    contraindications, 42
    for agitation in dementia, 20
    for COPD, 46–47
    treatment, 21*t*
thiazide diuretics, 66*t*
thyroid disorders, 3
torsemide, side effects, 66*t*
trazodone, 21, 23*t*

U

understimulation, 21*t*
urinary retention, 21*t*

V

valproate, 21
valsartan, side effects, 66*t*
valvular heart disease, 57
vascular dementia, 2
    frequency, 1*t*
    incidence of, 2
    treatment, 21*t*
vasodilators, adverse effects, 67*t*
ventilation, noninvasive, 49–50
ventilation/perfusion mismatch, 43
ventricular compliance, 57–58
Venturi masks, 43
vision loss, 21*t*
visual hallucinations, 18
vitamin B_{12} deficiency, 3
volume overload, 75

W

walkers, rolling, 45, 47
weight loss
    cholinesterase inhibitors and, 9
    COPD and, 51
    hospice eligibility and, 54
    unintential, 54
work effort, dyspnea and, 37